NEW

NURSING PHOTOBOOK

Providing Cardiovascular Care

NEW

NURSING PHOTOBOOK

Providing Cardiovascular Care

Springhouse Corporation
Springhouse, Pennsylvania

STAFF

Senior Publisher
Matthew Cahill

Clinical Manager
Cindy Tryniszewski, RN, MSN

Art Director
John Hubbard

Senior Editor
June Norris

Clinical Editors
Judith Schilling McCann, RN, BSN (clinical project editor), Beverly Tscheschlog, RN

Editor
Elizabeth Weinstein

Copy Editors
Cynthia C. Breuninger (manager), Lynette High, Doris Weinstock

Designers
Stephanie Peters (senior associate art director), Lorraine Carbo, Darcy Feralio

Photographer
John Gallagher

Typographers
Diane Paluba (manager), Elizabeth Bergman, Joyce Rossi Biletz, Phyllis Marron, Valerie Rosenberger

Manufacturing
Deborah Meiris (director), Pat Dorshaw (manager), T.A. Landis

Production Coordinator
Margaret A. Rastiello

Editorial Assistants
Beverly Lane, Mary Madden

Indexer
Barbara Hodgson

R A member of the Reed Elsevier plc group

PHOBK2-010795

Library of Congress Cataloging-in-Publication Data
Providing cardiovascular care.
    p. cm. — (New nursing photobooks)
Includes index.
    1. Cardiovascular system — Diseases — Nursing.
I. Springhouse Corporation.   II. Series
[DNLM: 1. Cardiovascular Diseases — nursing.
2. Monitoring, Physiologic — methods — nurses'
instruction.   WY 152.5 P969   1996 (P)]
RC674.76   1996
616.1 — dc20
DNLM/DLC   95-7924
ISBN 0-87434-809-9   CIP

CONTENTS

FOREWORD

In the last decade, major changes have occurred in cardiovascular care. As in many areas of nursing, cardiovascular care reflects advances in technology and treatments as well as evolving financial pressures. If you're an experienced nurse, you may remember a time when your main responsibility in caring for a patient after an acute myocardial infarction was to keep him from moving around too much during his 8 weeks of bed rest. But you probably know that in caring for an MI patient today, you're responsible for much more, including monitoring cardiac rhythms and administering complex drug therapy within a brief amount of time.

Today, more than ever before, you must develop, implement, and evaluate realistic plans of care based on a sound knowledge of current cardiovascular nursing care. If you practice in an outpatient care facility, your responsibility for identifying patients at risk for cardiovascular disease may involve performing a signal-averaged electrocardiogram (ECG). If you practice in an acute care setting, you must interpret, manage, and monitor a vast array of new technological devices. And if you're a cardiac rehabilitation nurse, you must be familiar with telemetry monitoring and be proficient at interpreting ECG rhythms—for example, differentiating between an aberrant and an ectopic rhythm.

As a busy nurse working in a demanding, ever-changing field, you must be able to rely on certain books as trusted companions. *Providing Cardiovascular Care* provides the versatility and comprehensive coverage you need. Written by nurses with years of patient care experience, this book *shows* you—in step-by-step photographs—every important technique for performing cardiac assessment and monitoring the cardiovascular system.

With over 350 photographs and an easy-to-use format, you can consult this book every day or once a week. The book begins with a section on assessing the heart and peripheral circulation and ends nearly 200 pages later with a section on monitoring left atrial pressure. *Providing Cardiovascular Care* puts both basic and highly complex information at your fingertips. The concise directions save you time. The clear, black-and-white close-up photographs provide the accuracy that's essential when you're trying to learn or brush up on a difficult technique. And when you're consulting a section on how to use the latest equipment, you can be confident that the information is current.

The book is divided into three major sections: "Assessing the Cardiovascular System," "Monitoring Cardiac Status," and "Monitoring Hemodynamic Status." Within these sections, you'll find thorough, step-by-step directions and accompanying photographs for 26 procedures or techniques.

"Monitoring Cardiac Status" begins with a discussion of electrocardiography, the ECG grid, and the electrical basis of the ECG. Following this are photostories—clear, concise explanations with photographs at every step—that explain how to perform hardwire and telemetry monitoring, a 12-lead ECG, a signal-averaged ECG, and ST-segment monitoring.

"Monitoring Hemodynamic Status" ranges from how to set up transducers and manage an arterial and a pulmonary artery line to how to monitor central venous pressure, perform thermodilution monitoring, and monitor left atrial pressure.

Throughout the text, graphic devices, called logos, help you quickly locate important information. *Clinical tips* alert you to more efficient or alternative steps in many procedures. *Insights and interpretations* guides your interpretation of physical findings and test results—for instance, discussing how to read rhythm strips and showing you examples. *Complications* charts provide information about patient risks in certain procedures (for instance, managing arterial lines), including signs and symptoms, possible causes, how to intervene, and how to prevent such complications. *Troubleshooting* charts help you recognize and respond to alarms, abnormal waveforms and pressures, and other equipment problems.

Staying current in the complex, changing field of cardiovascular care isn't easy, and you might often wish for an expert at your side. Now you can have one. By providing you with quick access to a wealth of information, *Providing Cardiovascular Care* is like having a trusted, experienced nurse you can consult any hour of the day. This book is a must if you want to update and expand your knowledge of cardiovascular care.

Kristine A. Bludau Scordo, RN, PhD
 Clinical Director
 Clinical Nurse Specialist
 Cardiology Center of Cincinnati

Assessing the Cardiovascular System

EXAMINING THE HEART

In North America, heart disease represents the leading cause of death and debility. That's one compelling reason for you to make your cardiac assessment thorough and precise. Before beginning, however, make sure that you're familiar with cardiac anatomy and physiology. (See *Cardiac position*, below, and *Cardiac structures and function*, page 4.)

Then assess the patient's history and chief complaints. (See *Exploring cardiac complaints*, page 5.) Continue with the examination that appears on the following pages featuring the essential components and techniques of cardiac assessment.

Cardiac position

As you perform a cardiac assessment, keep in mind the heart's location in the chest and its relationship to other organs.

Bony thoracic structures (the sternum and the ribs) protect the heart where it lies obliquely in the chest, with about two-thirds of it located to the left of the sternum. The base of the heart corresponds to the level of the third costal cartilage. Normally, the apex of the heart lies at the fifth left intercostal space, at the midclavicular line. The right end of the inferior surface lies under the sixth or seventh chondrosternal junction. Within the chest, the lungs surround the heart laterally and superiorly. The esophagus lies posterior to the heart; the diaphragm, inferior to it.

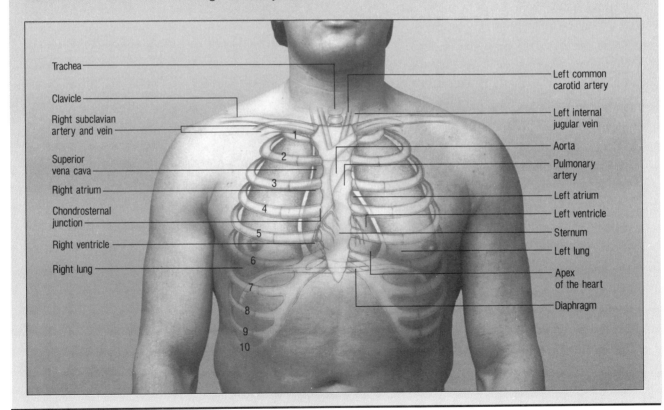

Trachea

Clavicle

Right subclavian
artery and vein

Superior
vena cava

Right atrium

Chondrosternal
junction

Right ventricle

Right lung

Left common
carotid artery

Left internal
jugular vein

Aorta

Pulmonary
artery

Left atrium

Left ventricle

Sternum

Left lung

Apex
of the heart

Diaphragm

Contributors to this section include *Sandra J. Bixler, RN, MSN, CCRN*, a cardiac clinical nurse specialist at Reading Hospital and Medical Center, Wyomissing, Pa., and *Teresa A. Palmer, RN, MSN, CANP,* a nurse practitioner in adult cardiac surgery at Robert Wood Johnson University Hospital, New Brunswick, N.J. The publisher thanks *Hill-Rom,* Batesville, Ind., for its help.

Cardiac structures and function

As you assess the heart, keep in mind how cardiac anatomy contributes to the heart's central role as a pump, circulating life-sustaining blood to the body's organs and tissues.

Structures

Cardiac structures include the pericardium, three layers of the heart wall, four chambers, and four valves. The pericardium, a closed sac, surrounds the heart and great vessels. The pericardium has an inner (visceral) layer that forms the epicardium and an outer (parietal) layer. The pericardial space between these two layers normally contains from 10 to 20 ml of serous fluid, allowing the epicardium to glide smoothly without friction during heart muscle contraction and relaxation.

The heart wall consists of three layers: endocardium, myocardium, and epicardium. The endocardium (the inner layer) provides a smooth surface for the inner heart structures. The myocardium (the thick middle layer) is made of muscle fibers responsible for contraction. The epicardium forms the thin outermost layer.

The heart chambers include the right and left atria and the right and left ventricles. Heart valves include the atrioventricular (tricuspid and mitral) and the semilunar (pulmonic and aortic) valves. Located at the right atrioventricular orifice, the tricuspid valve consists of three triangular cusps. Located at the left atrioventricular opening, the mitral valve consists of two cusps. Positioned at the orifices of the pulmonary artery and the aorta, the two semilunar valves have three cusps each.

Function

The chambers and valves work together guiding blood through the heart. The arrows in the illustration below indicate the direction of blood flow. The right side of the heart, which includes the right atrium and right ventricle, receives venous blood from the body and pumps it to the lungs for oxygenation. The left side of the heart, which contains the left atrium and left ventricle, receives oxygenated blood from the lungs and pumps it to all body tissues. Blood exits the left ventricle through the aortic valve.

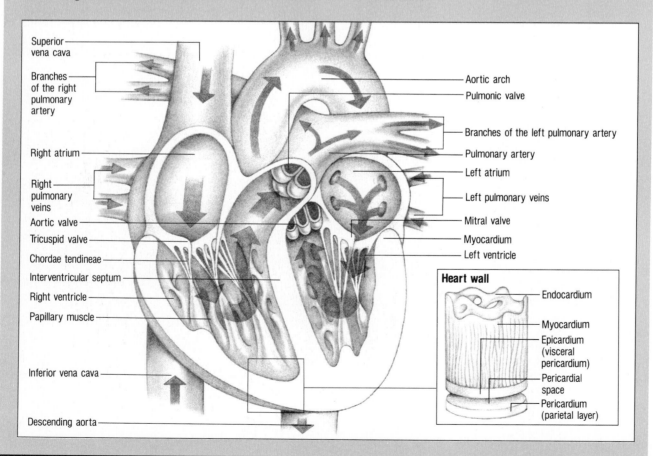

Exploring cardiac complaints

Begin your assessment of the patient's chief complaint by investigating his cardiac health history. Ask the patient why he's seeking medical care. Document his answer in his own words.

If the patient has a medical complaint, ask how long he's had the problem and when it began. Explore any associated signs and symptoms. If he reports chest pain, ask about the pain's location, radiation, intensity, and duration. Also ask about precipitating, exacerbating, and relieving factors. If the patient is experiencing chest pain during the assessment, obtain as accurate a description as possible.

As you interview the patient and compile assessment data, remember to avoid leading questions and to use familiar expressions rather than medical terms. If the patient isn't in distress, ask open-ended questions, which require more than a yes-or-no response. Simultaneously, perform the physical examination, proceeding from inspection and palpation through percussion and auscultation.

Use the following questions to help your patient accurately describe his cardiovascular symptoms.
- [ ] Where in your chest do you feel pain?
- [ ] Can you point to the site of your pain? Does it radiate to any other areas?
- [ ] Do you get a burning or squeezing sensation in your chest?
- [ ] How long have you been having chest pain? How long does an attack last?
- [ ] What relieves the pain?
- [ ] How would you rate the intensity of your pain on a scale of 1 to 10, with 10 as the most severe pain?
- [ ] Do you ever feel short of breath? Does a particular body position seem to bring this on? Which one? How long does any shortness of breath last? What relieves it?
- [ ] Has breathing trouble ever awakened you from sleep?
- [ ] Do you ever wake up coughing? How often?
- [ ] Have you ever coughed up blood?
- [ ] Does your heart ever pound, race, or skip a beat? If so, when does this happen?
- [ ] Do you ever feel dizzy or faint? What seems to bring this on?
- [ ] Do your feet or ankles swell? At what time of day? What, if anything, relieves the swelling?
- [ ] Do you urinate more frequently at night?
- [ ] Do any activities easily tire you? Which ones? Have you had to limit your activities or rest more often while doing them? Does rest relieve the fatigue?

Inspecting the jugular veins

You'll need only your stethoscope, a light source, a centimeter ruler, and a warm, quiet, private setting with adequate lighting. Wash your hands and explain the procedure to the patient. Begin by observing the jugular veins to detect distention. Assist the patient into semi-Fowler's position. Turn his head slightly away from the side you're examining. Angle the light source (a penlight, for example) to cast shadows along the neck. (The shadows will help you see pulse wave motion.) Measure the level of distention in fingerbreadths above the clavicle.

▶ *Clinical tip:* You'll see jugular vein distention only if the patient has right ventricular dysfunction.

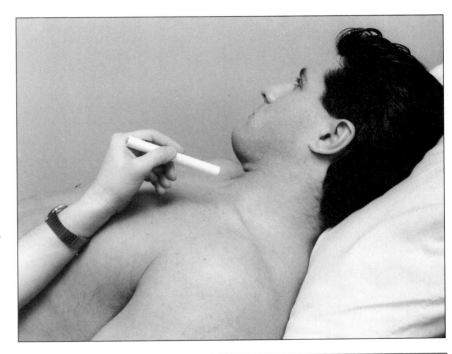

With the patient in the same position, estimate central venous pressure. Begin by palpating the clavicles where they join the sternum (the suprasternal notch). Place your fingers here and slide them down the sternum until you feel a bony protuberance, known as the angle of Louis (or the sternal angle). Place a centimeter ruler vertically (perpendicular to the chest) at this angle. From the ruler, extend a sturdy square-cornered piece of paper horizontally along the highest level of venous pulsation (as shown). Normally, venous pressure is seen below the angle of Louis or less than 4 cm above it.

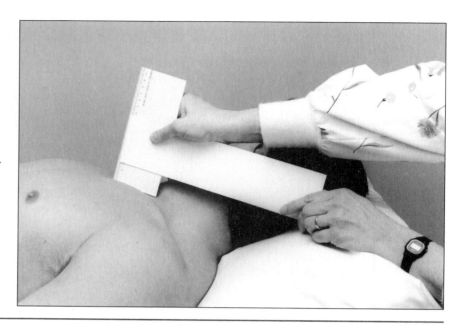

Inspecting the precordium

Have the patient sit on the examination table or stand with his chest exposed so you can inspect his chest and identify the necessary anatomic landmarks.

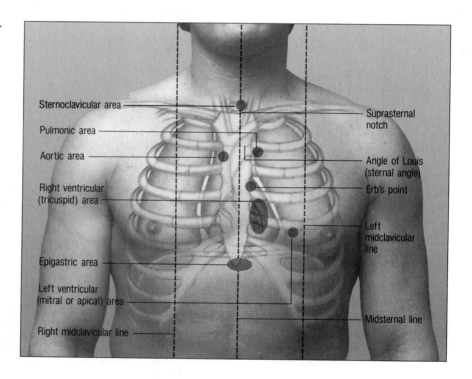

Sternoclavicular area

Pulmonic area

Aortic area

Right ventricular (tricuspid) area

Epigastric area

Left ventricular (mitral or apical) area

Right midclavicular line

Suprasternal notch

Angle of Louis (sternal angle)

Erb's point

Left midclavicular line

Midsternal line

To see lateral landmarks, have the patient raise his arms over his head.

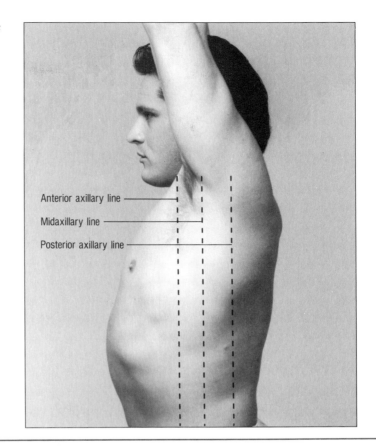

Anterior axillary line
Midaxillary line
Posterior axillary line

Help the patient into the supine position. If he can't tolerate this position, raise his head slightly. Standing by his side—usually his right side—mentally note the anatomic landmarks. Then position the light source (your penlight or gooseneck lamp, for example) so that it again provides indirect light. You should see shadows across the patient's chest. These will help you detect cardiac pulsations.

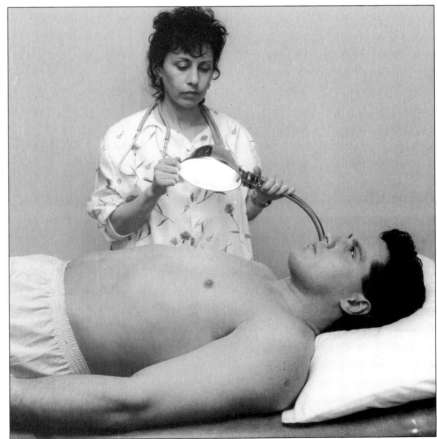

Observe the patient's chest for the apical impulse (pulsations at the apex of the heart). This normally appears in the fifth intercostal space at, or just medial to, the left midclavicular line (left ventricular area). This impulse reflects the location and size of the left ventricle. It usually occupies only one intercostal space.

▶ *Clinical tip:* If a female patient has large breasts, displace them so that you can see the apical impulse. If a patient's chest is enlarged from obesity or emphysema, have him sit up. This position enhances pulsations.

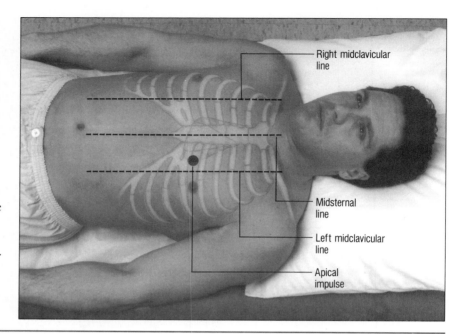

Right midclavicular line

Midsternal line

Left midclavicular line

Apical impulse

Palpating the precordium

Palpate the apical impulse in the left ventricular area. Place your fingertips or the ball of your hand (the palmar surface at the base of the fingers) at the fifth intercostal space, left midclavicular line. This is called the point of maximum impulse (PMI). Light palpation should reveal a tap with each heartbeat. If palpation discloses a weak, an unusually forceful, or a displaced apical impulse, notify the doctor. These are abnormal findings.

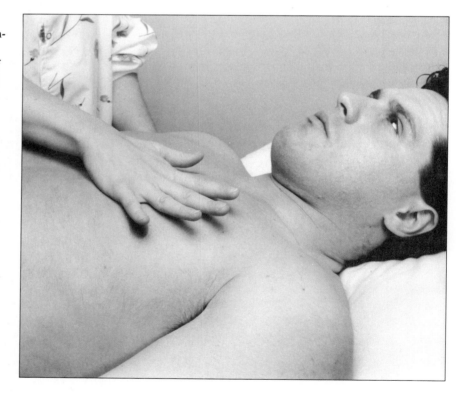

Systematically palpate the sterno-clavicular, aortic, pulmonic, and right ventricular areas for pulsations. Normally, pulsations aren't palpable in these areas. However, in some patients, palpation reveals a vibration that feels like a cat purring. These sensations are heart murmurs (or thrills).

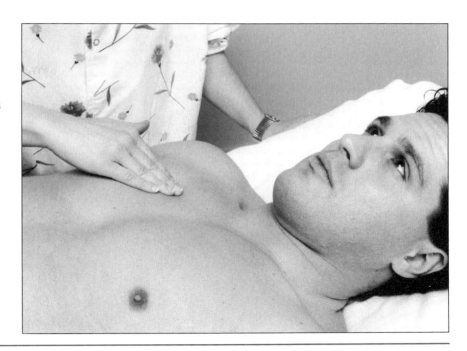

Percussing the precordium

To judge heart size, percuss the heart's borders. Begin at the anterior left axillary line, and percuss toward the sternum in the fifth intercostal space. Note the changes from resonance to dullness (usually near the PMI). If the border extends to the midclavicular line, the left ventricle may be enlarged. On the chest's right side, the heart lies under the sternum and can't be percussed.

▷ ***Clinical tip:*** If possible, refer to the patient's chest X-ray, which reliably reveals heart size.

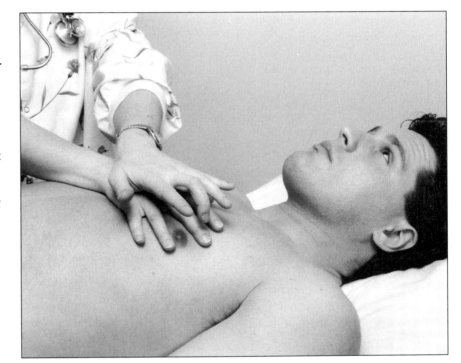

Auscultating the heart

Keep the patient covered and supine, with his head level or slightly elevated. Expose the area to be auscultated. Then warm your stethoscope between your hands (as shown). Have the patient inhale normally through his nose and exhale by mouth.

▶ *Clinical tip:* Don't auscultate through clothing or dressings, which block sound. Also avoid extra noise by keeping the stethoscope tubing off the patient's body or other surfaces.

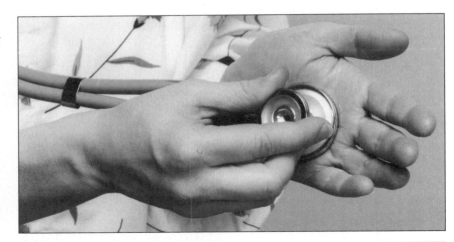

To measure the apical pulse rate, place the diaphragm of the stethoscope over the PMI. Then count the heartbeats for 1 minute.

▶ *Clinical tip:* Note the heart rhythm during this time. Is it regular or irregular? If it's irregular, does the rhythm have a pattern? If so, note the pattern.

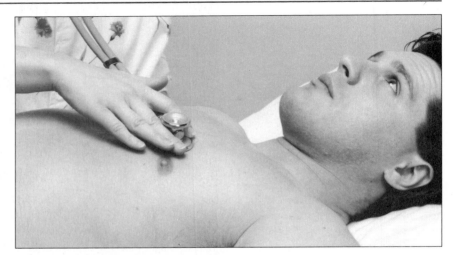

Auscultating normal heart sounds

Mentally identify the four cardiac auscultation sites (shown here in the upright, frontal view to aid visualization). Listen at each site in this sequence: aortic area (second intercostal space, right sternal border), pulmonic area (second intercostal space, left sternal border), mitral area (fifth intercostal space, midclavicular line), and tricuspid area (fifth intercostal space, left sternal border). Because the opening and closing of the heart valves create most normal heart sounds, auscultation sites lie close together in the chest, behind or to the left of the sternum. Auscultation sites are not located directly over the valves; they lie over the pathways the blood takes as it flows through them.

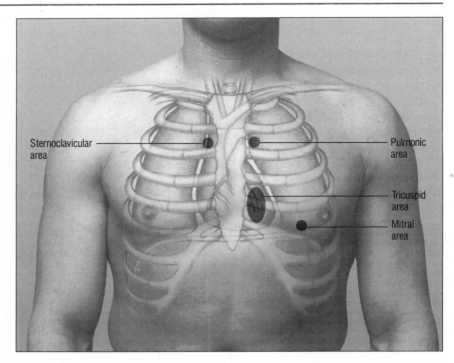

With the patient still supine, place the diaphragm of the stethoscope on one of the auscultation sites. Listen to several cardiac cycles to become familiar with the rate and rhythm of S$_1$ and S$_2$. Normal heart sounds last a fraction of a second and are followed by slightly longer silences. Listen closely to these sounds. Their timing in the cardiac cycle tells you how well each valve works.

▶ **Clinical tip:** Always identify S$_1$ and S$_2$ first because you need to be familiar with normal sounds before you can identify abnormal ones.

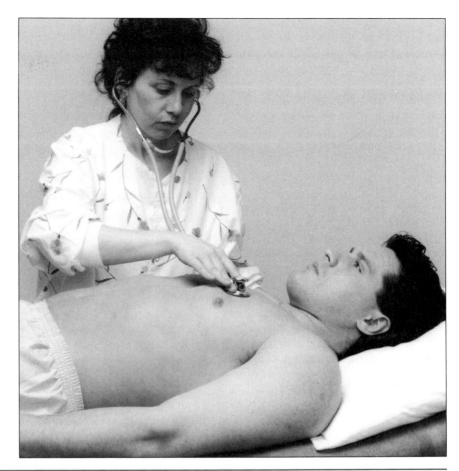

Once you're familiar with the rate and rhythm of normal heart sounds, listen for the heart sounds in each of the four areas following the sequence described previously. First, pressing firmly, use the diaphragm of the stethoscope (as shown). Then, pressing lightly, use the bell.

Note: In the aortic area (shown) and the pulmonic area, S$_1$ is normally quieter than S$_2$. A split S$_2$ may be heard during inspiration in the pulmonic area. In the tricuspid and mitral areas, S$_1$ is normally louder than S$_2$. A split S$_2$ may be heard in the tricuspid area.

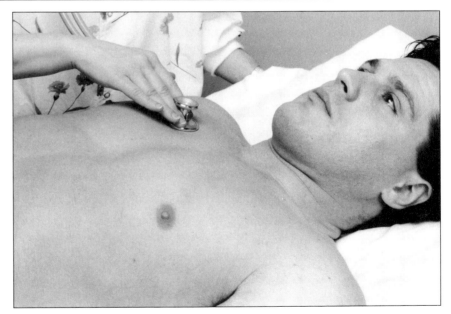

If you have difficulty distinguishing S_1 from S_2, try palpating the carotid artery as you auscultate. S_1 occurs almost simultaneously with the beat of the carotid pulse.

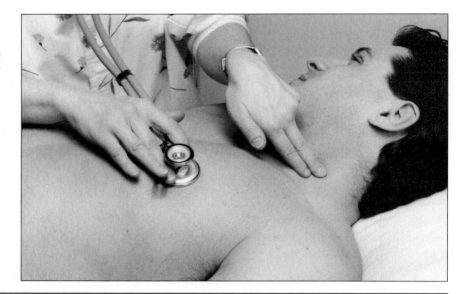

Alternatively or additionally, you can listen to heart sounds with the patient in a left lateral recumbent position. Although S_1 and S_2 are clearly heard with the patient in this position, you'll find this position best for auscultating low-pitched sounds associated with atrioventricular problems, such as mitral valve murmurs and extra heart sounds. To detect these sounds, place the bell over the apical area.

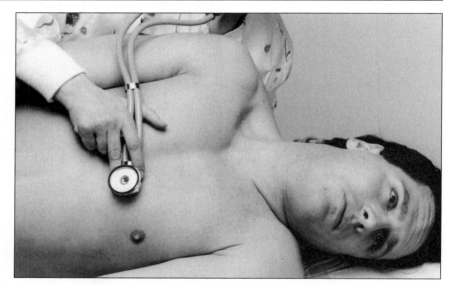

Another alternative or additional way to hear heart sounds is to place the patient in the forward-leaning position. With the patient in this position, you can clearly hear not only normal sounds but also high-pitched sounds related to semilunar valve problems, such as aortic and pulmonic valve murmurs.

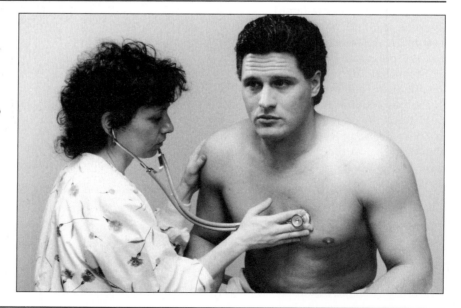

Auscultating additional heart sounds

When auscultating for S_1 and S_2, you may hear additional heart sounds: S_3, S_4, or both. Listen for S_3 (also called a ventricular gallop) when the patient is in the left lateral recumbent position. Place the bell of the stethoscope at the tricuspid and mitral areas. Expect to hear S_3 during early to mid-diastole, just after S_2, at the end of ventricular filling. If the right ventricle is noncompliant, you'll hear the sound in the tricuspid area; if the left ventricle is noncompliant, you'll hear the sound in the mitral area.

▶ *Clinical tip:* The rhythm of S_3 resembles a horse galloping; its cadence resembles the word *ken-tuc-ky* or *lub-dub-by.*

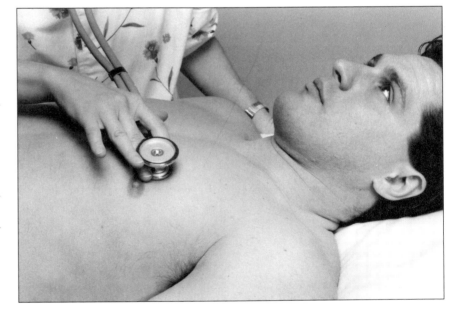

Listen for S_4 (also called atrial or presystolic gallop) with the patient in the supine position. Place the bell of the stethoscope on the patient's chest over the tricuspid and mitral areas. Expect to hear this heart sound late in diastole, immediately before the S_1 of the next cycle. S_4 is associated with the acceleration and deceleration of blood entering a chamber that resists additional filling. In right ventricular dysfunction, you'll hear S_4 in the tricuspid area; in left ventricular dysfunction, you'll hear it in the mitral area.

▶ *Clinical tip:* S_4 has the same cadence as the word *tennes-see* or *le-lub-dub.*

To detect a pericardial friction rub, have the patient sit upright and lean forward or exhale. This enhances the sound of the friction rub. Then use the diaphragm of the stethoscope to auscultate at the third left intercostal space along the lower left sternal border. Listen for a harsh, scratchy, scraping or squeaking sound.

▶ *Clinical tip:* If possible, have the patient hold his breath for a few seconds while you listen. This can eliminate noisy respiratory sounds that may interfere with auscultating for rubs. A rub usually indicates pericarditis.

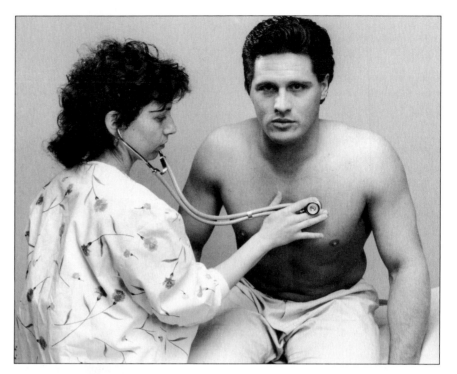

To detect a carotid artery bruit, auscultate each carotid artery by lightly placing the bell of the stethoscope over the carotid artery—first on one side of the trachea, then on the other side. Normally, you should hear no vascular sounds. If you detect a blowing, swishing sound, this usually indicates turbulent blood flow, which may occur in persons who have cardiovascular disease.

▶ *Clinical tip:* Ask the patient to hold his breath, if he can. This will eliminate respiratory sounds that may interfere with your findings.

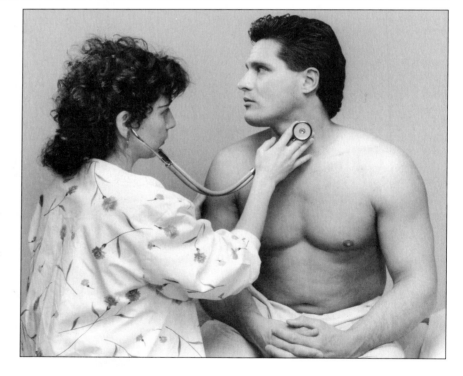

Understanding normal heart sounds in the cardiac cycle

The cardiac cycle has two phases: systole, when the ventricles contract, increasing blood pressure and ejecting blood into the aorta and the pulmonary artery; and diastole, when the ventricles relax and blood pressure decreases, thereby contracting the atria. Using your stethoscope, you can hear each phase reverberate distinctively as the heart's valves open and close.

Sounds of systole

At the beginning of systole, increasing ventricular pressure forces the mitral and tricuspid valves to shut. The closing of these atrioventricular (AV) valves produces the first heart sound (S_1), or the *lub* of *lub-dub*. The ventricular pressure builds until it exceeds that in the pulmonary artery and the aorta. Then the aortic and pulmonic (semilunar) valves open and the ventricles eject blood into the arteries (see arrows below).

Sounds of diastole

As the ventricles empty and relax, ventricular pressure falls below that in the pulmonary artery and the aorta. The semilunar valves close, producing the second heart sound (S_2), or the *dub* of *lub-dub,* and marking the end of systole. As the ventricles relax during diastole, the pressure in the ventricles is less than that in the atria. The AV valves open, and blood begins to flow into the ventricles from the atria (see arrows below). When the ventricles become full near the end of diastole, the atria contract to send the rest of the blood to the ventricles. Ventricular pressure is now greater than atrial pressure. The AV valves close, marking the beginning of systole and repetition of the cardiac cycle.

Note: Events on the right side of the heart occur a fraction of a second after events on the left side because the pressure is lower on the right side of the heart.

Systole

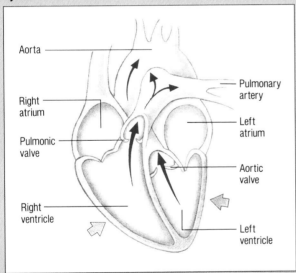

Aorta
Right atrium
Pulmonic valve
Right ventricle
Pulmonary artery
Left atrium
Aortic valve
Left ventricle

Diastole

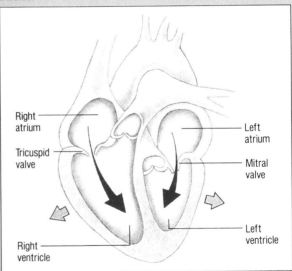

Right atrium
Tricuspid valve
Right ventricle
Left atrium
Mitral valve
Left ventricle

Recognizing abnormal heart sounds

Whenever auscultation reveals an abnormal heart sound, you'll need to identify the sound and its timing in the cardiac cycle. Knowing these characteristics helps you identify the possible cause as described in the chart below.

ABNORMAL HEART SOUND	CYCLICAL TIMING	POSSIBLE CAUSES
Accentuated S_1	Beginning of systole	Mitral stenosis; fever
Diminished S_1	Beginning of systole	Mitral regurgitation; severe mitral regurgitation with calcified, immobile valve; heart block
Split S_1	Beginning of systole	Right bundle-branch block
Accentuated S_2	End of systole	Pulmonary or systemic hypertension
Diminished or inaudible S_2	End of systole	Aortic or pulmonic stenosis
Persistent S_2 split	End of systole	Delayed closure of the pulmonic valve, usually from overfilling of the right ventricle, causing prolonged systolic ejection time
Reversed or paradoxical S_2 split that appears in expiration and disappears in inspiration	End of systole	Delayed ventricular stimulation; left bundle-branch block or prolonged left ventricular ejection time
S_3 (ventricular gallop)	Early diastole	Overdistention of ventricles in rapid-filling segment of diastole; mitral insufficiency or ventricular failure (normal in children and young adults)
S_4 (atrial or presystolic gallop)	Late diastole	Forceful atrial contraction from resistance to ventricular filling late in diastole (resulting from left ventricular hypertrophy), pulmonic stenosis, hypertension, coronary artery disease, or aortic stenosis
Pericardial friction rub (grating or leathery sound at left sternal border; usually muffled, high-pitched, and transient)	Throughout systole and diastole	Pericardial inflammation

EXAMINING PERIPHERAL CIRCULATION

Because assessing your patient's peripheral vascular system provides information about blood circulation through the arteries, veins, and capillaries, you'll need to be familiar with the major vessels and pulse points before you begin your assessment. (See *Vascular structures.*)

Vascular structures

Below are the major arteries (red), veins (gray), and pulse points of the vascular system.

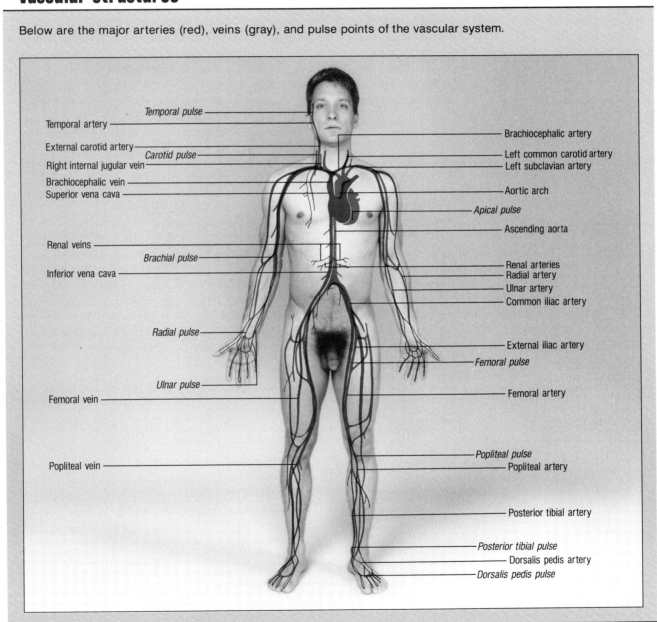

Temporal pulse
Temporal artery
External carotid artery
Carotid pulse
Right internal jugular vein
Brachiocephalic vein
Superior vena cava
Renal veins
Brachial pulse
Inferior vena cava
Radial pulse
Ulnar pulse
Femoral vein
Popliteal vein

Brachiocephalic artery
Left common carotid artery
Left subclavian artery
Aortic arch
Apical pulse
Ascending aorta
Renal arteries
Radial artery
Ulnar artery
Common iliac artery
External iliac artery
Femoral pulse
Femoral artery
Popliteal pulse
Popliteal artery
Posterior tibial artery
Posterior tibial pulse
Dorsalis pedis artery
Dorsalis pedis pulse

Lynne Patzek Miller, RN,C, BS, operating room manager at Doylestown (Pa.) Hospital, and *Teresa A. Palmer, RN, MSN, CANP,* a nurse practitioner in adult cardiac surgery at Robert Wood Johnson University Hospital, New Brunswick, N.J., contributed to this section. The publisher thanks *Hill-Rom,* Batesville, Ind., and *North Penn Hospital,* Lansdale, Pa., for their help.

REVIEWING THE VASCULAR SYSTEM

A vast network of blood vessels, the vascular system keeps blood circulating to and from every functioning cell in the body. This core network consists of arteries and veins and such extensions as capillaries.

The arteries carry oxygenated blood from the lungs to the heart and then to the body. The only artery that doesn't carry oxygenated blood is the pulmonary artery.

The main artery—the aorta—branches into vessels that supply specific organs or areas of the body. Three major branches arise from the arch of the aorta: the left common carotid, left subclavian, and left brachiocephalic arteries. These vessels take oxygen to the brain, arms, and upper chest. The descending aorta takes oxygen to GI and genitourinary organs, the spinal column, and the lower chest and abdominal muscles. From the abdominal area, the aorta forks into the iliac arteries, which further branch into the femoral arteries.

To complete the cycle, the venous system returns blood to the heart and then to the lungs for gas exchange and reoxygenation. The only vein that carries oxygenated blood is the pulmonary vein.

ASSESSING CIRCULATION

Your assessment of peripheral circulation typically begins as you take the patient's pulse. You can feel or hear the pressure wave of blood exiting the heart and surging through the arteries. Normally, you can palpate this recurring fluid wave—or pulse—at locations on the body where an artery crosses over bone or firm tissue. By assessing peripheral pulses, you can indirectly determine the status of peripheral arterial circulation.

To evaluate the peripheral vasculature, you'll perform inspection, palpation, and auscultation—with palpation as the primary tool for assessing blood flow to the extremities. To palpate pulses safely, apply gentle pressure to each pulse with the index and middle fingers of your dominant hand. Document the rate (beats/minute), rhythm (regular or irregular), amplitude (strength of contractions), and bilateral symmetry of each pulse.

One of the most telling signs of peripheral vascular health or disease is pulse amplitude—especially in such areas as the neck, arms, and legs. This sign reflects the vigor of left ventricular contractions and the patency of peripheral vessels. To evaluate pulse amplitude, use a numerical scale, a descriptive term, or another system favored by your hospital. The following numerical scale and the corresponding descriptions of pulse amplitude are in common use:

+3 — bounding (readily palpable, forceful, not easily obliterated by finger pressure)
+2 — normal (easily palpable and obliterated only by strong finger pressure)
+1 — weak or thready (hard to palpate and easily obliterated by slight finger pressure)
0 — absent (undiscernible).

Remember, only +2 describes a normal pulse.

To complement your physical assessment findings, you'll need to take a thorough health history. Ask the patient about factors that can significantly affect peripheral circulation. For example, ask about his job requirements, activities of daily living, and cardiovascular health and whether he has a history of diabetes. (See *Exploring circulatory complaints.*)

 ASSESSMENT CHECKLIST

Exploring circulatory complaints

To detect potential abnormalities in peripheral circulation, conduct a thorough health history. If you think the patient's peripheral circulation may be impaired or if he voices related complaints, ask questions to elicit further information, as follows:

☐ Do you have a history of heart disease? If so, can you describe the problem?

☐ Do you have high blood pressure?

☐ Have you ever been diagnosed with an aortic aneurysm?

☐ Do you have a history of diabetes? If so, how long have you had it? Can you describe your treatment plan?

☐ Do your shoes or rings ever feel tight? Do your ankles or feet ever swell? If so, when does this occur?

☐ Have you noticed any change in feeling in your legs? If so, would you describe this feeling as numbness or pain? How long does this feeling last?

☐ Have you noticed any change in color in your legs or feet? If so, can you describe the change? When does it occur and how long does it last?

☐ Do you have any sores or ulcers on your legs or feet? If so, are they healing?

☐ What kinds of activities does your job require? Do your job duties include much standing or sitting in one place?

Preparing to assess peripheral circulation

Begin by assembling your equipment: gloves and a stethoscope.

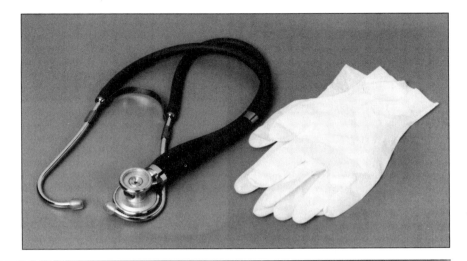

Wash your hands. Explain the procedure to the patient, answer any questions he may have, and provide reassurance. Then place him in a comfortable, relaxed position. Use the supine position if he can tolerate it: This position gives you easy access to all peripheral pulses.

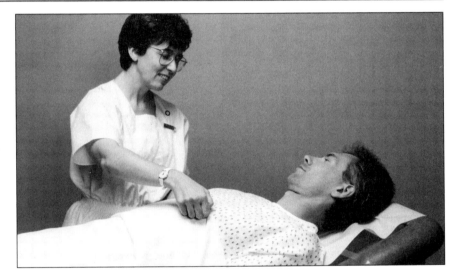

Inspecting the arms and legs

Observe the patient's arms and legs. Note the color of his skin (pink, pale, or cyanotic), and check closely for edema. If you observe edema, identify its location and check for symmetry. Note the location and size of any lesions, rashes, or scaly areas. Also assess hair patterns on the arms, legs, hands, and feet. (The presence of hair indicates an adequate arterial blood supply.)

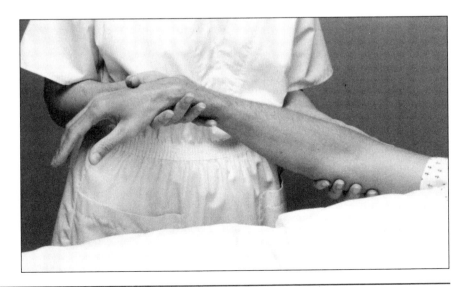

Observe the nail beds for normal growth. Note any thickening of the nails, an indicator of impaired circulation.

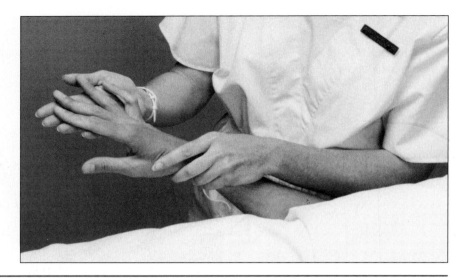

Palpating peripheral pulses

Palpate the skin on the arms and legs to determine its temperature (cold, cool, warm, or hot).

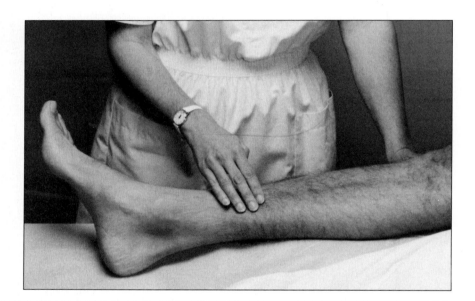

If you noticed any edema during inspection, determine its type (pitting or nonpitting) and degree (from +1 to +4). To do so, press the area firmly with your finger for 5 to 10 seconds, and then remove your finger. Note the extent and duration of a depression on the skin.

▶ *Clinical tip:* Pitting edema progresses in severity from +1 (a barely perceptible depression) to +4 (a persistent pit as deep as 1″ [2.5 cm]). The higher the score, the more significant the edema.

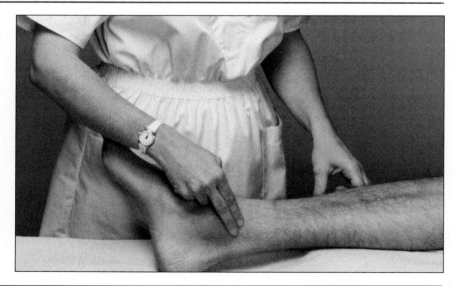

Squeeze the nail beds on all extremities to produce blanching. Note how much time passes before the nail bed color returns.
▷ **Clinical tip:** Normal capillary refill time is 3 seconds or less.

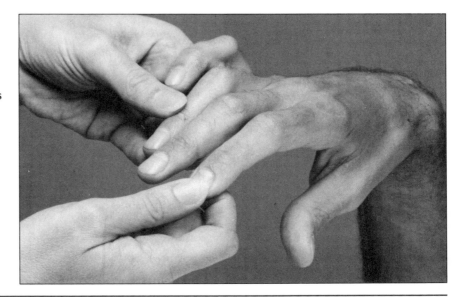

Next, palpate the peripheral pulses, beginning with the carotid pulse. Place your fingers lightly on the patient's neck just medial to the trachea and below the jaw angle (as shown). Repeat the action on the opposite side.
▷ **Clinical tip:** Palpate only one carotid artery at a time; simultaneous palpation can slow the pulse or decrease the blood pressure, causing the patient to faint.

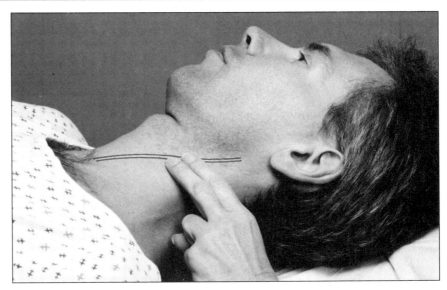

To palpate the brachial pulse, position your fingers in the groove between the biceps and the triceps muscle, just above the elbow. Repeat the action on the opposite arm.

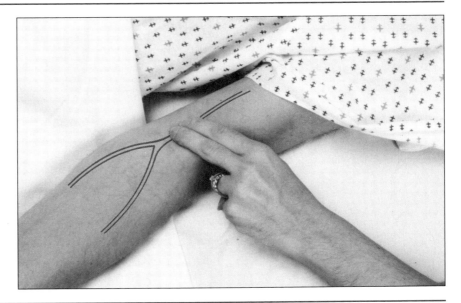

To palpate the radial pulse, place your fingers on the medial and ventral side of the wrist, in line with the thumb (as shown). Repeat the action on the opposite wrist.

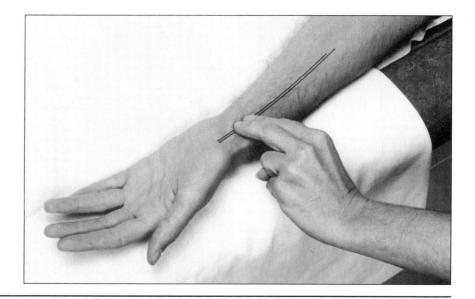

To palpate the femoral pulse, put on gloves, and press deeply about midway between the anterior superior iliac spine and the symphysis pubis (as shown). Repeat the action on the opposite side. (Then remove the gloves if you wish.)

▶ **Clinical tip:** In obese patients, palpate the crease of the groin, halfway between the pubic bone and the hip bone.

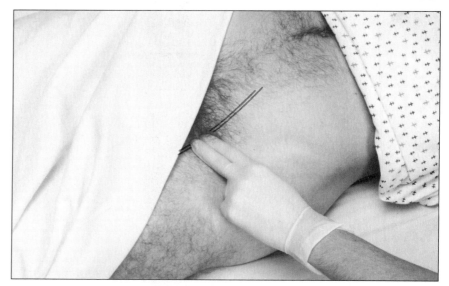

To palpate the popliteal pulse, flex the patient's knee. Press the fingers of both hands deeply into the popliteal fossa at the back of the knee. Repeat the action on the opposite knee.

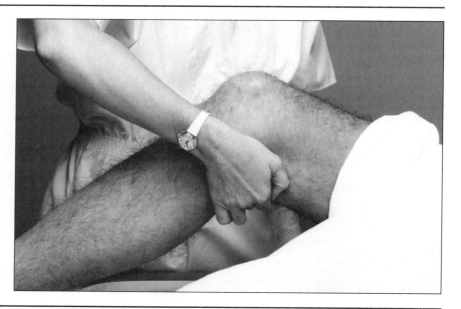

If you can't palpate the popliteal pulse with the patient in the position described above, reposition him onto his abdomen (if he can tolerate this position). Press deeply into the popliteal fossa to palpate the pulse (as shown).

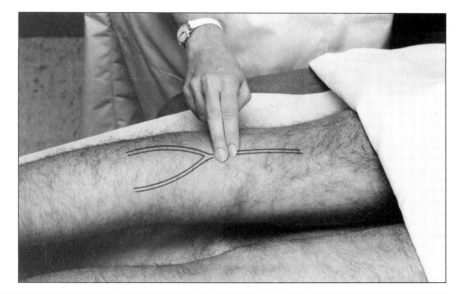

To palpate the posterior tibial pulse, apply pressure slightly below the medial malleolus of the ankle. Repeat the action on the opposite ankle.

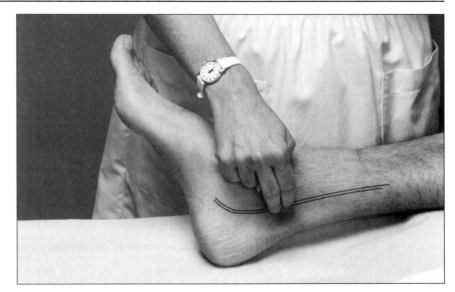

To palpate the dorsalis pedis pulse, position your fingers in the medial dorsum of the foot, just lateral to the extensor tendon of the great toe. If the pulse is difficult to palpate, instruct the patient to point his toes downward. Repeat the action on the opposite foot.

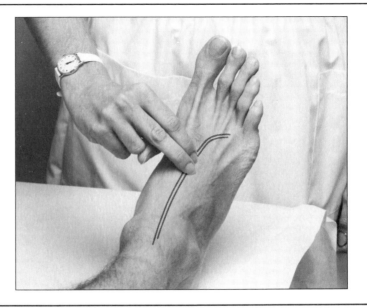

Auscultating peripheral pulses with a stethoscope

If you can locate peripheral pulses with palpation alone, proceed to auscultate blood flow with a stethoscope. Place the bell of the stethoscope over the carotid artery (as shown), and ask the patient to hold his breath. Listen for vascular sounds (such as murmurs or bruits). Repeat the action on the opposite side. Normally, you should hear no vascular sounds over the peripheral arteries. Vascular sounds in these areas may indicate a central circulation problem.

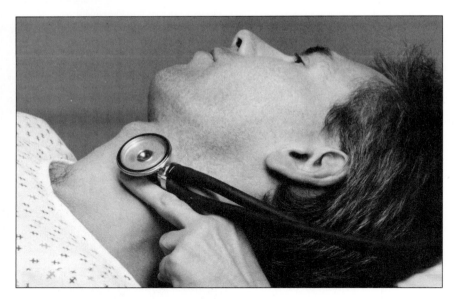

After putting on gloves, locate the femoral artery and place the bell of the stethoscope over the site. Listen for vascular sounds; then repeat the action on the opposite side. (Afterward, you may remove the gloves if you wish.)

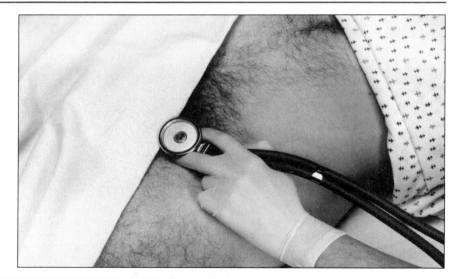

Place the bell of the stethoscope over the popliteal pulse site. Listen for vascular sounds. Repeat the action on the opposite side.

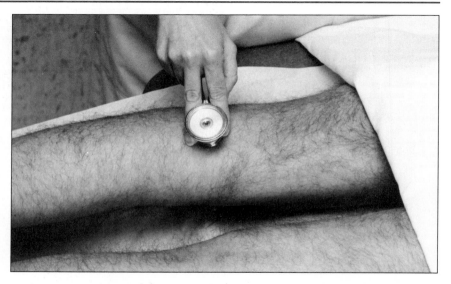

Auscultating peripheral pulses with ultrasound

If you can't locate peripheral pulses by palpation alone, use a Doppler ultrasound stethoscope to locate pulses and auscultate blood flow. Apply a small amount of coupling gel (not water-soluble lubricant) to the area being assessed and on the head of the ultrasound transducer (a sensitive wandlike component that amplifies the sound of blood flowing through the vessels and that can convert ultrasonic waves to electrical impulses).

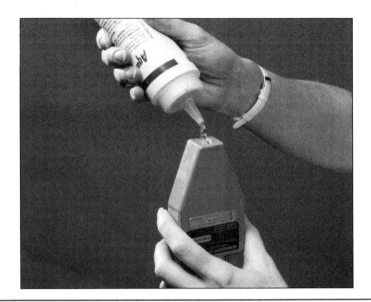

Turn the volume-control knob counterclockwise to the lowest audible setting while depressing the ON button (as shown). Adjust the volume so that you receive a clear amplification of the pulse.

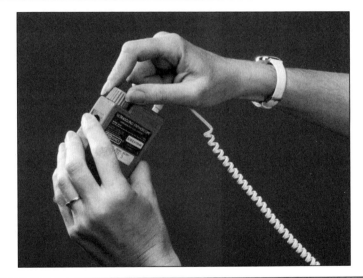

Position the transducer on the skin directly over the selected artery. Then angle the transducer about 45 degrees from the artery, making sure that the gel comes between the skin and the transducer. Move the transducer slowly in a circular motion until you locate the center of the artery. This positioning will help you obtain a clear, pulsating sound.

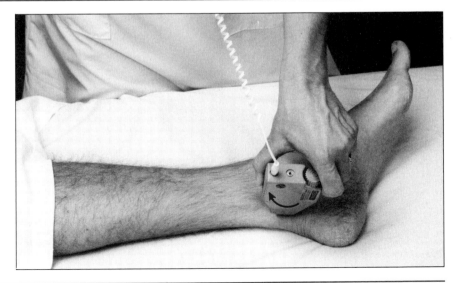

Count the signals for 60 seconds to determine the pulse rate. Wipe away any gel from the pulse site with a gauze pad, and mark the spots where you heard the pulse. This will help you relocate the pulse if necessary.

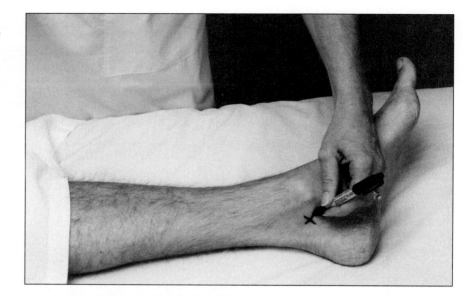

Then clean the head of the transducer with a clean gauze pad. Document all findings on the patient's assessment flow sheet. Report any abnormal findings to the doctor.

▶ *Clinical tip:* When cleaning the head of the transducer, don't use alcohol or an abrasive cleaner. These substances can damage the head, interfering with sound transmission.

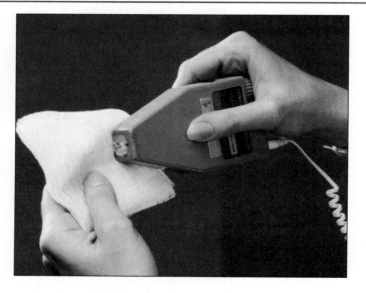

Monitoring Cardiac Status

LEARNING ABOUT CARDIAC MONITORING

When patients die from acute myocardial infarction, arrhythmias are the most common culprit. These cardiac disturbances usually result from thrombi or from an abrupt increase in myocardial oxygen demand. To identify arrhythmias promptly and allow early treatment, you can use cardiac monitoring. Such monitoring allows continuous evaluation of the heart's electrical activity.

Patients with arrhythmias aren't the only ones who may need cardiac monitoring. The procedure is commonly performed after major surgery and chest trauma. It's also performed for patients with severe electrolyte disturbances, major organ failure, and hemodynamic instability.

Besides providing clues that help you determine the patient's underlying problem, continuous cardiac monitoring helps you select the most appropriate intervention. What's more, it helps you evaluate the effects of therapy.

ELECTROCARDIOGRAPHY

The basis for cardiac monitoring is electrocardiography (ECG)—a representation on the body's surface of the heart's electrical activity (see *Understanding the ECG grid*, page 30). Although the ECG portrays this electrical activity, its appearance also depends on the sequence of electrical activation by the heart's chambers, the adequacy of the blood supply to the heart muscle, and the ability of the conducting system to initiate and transmit the electrical impulse.

The electrical activity produces a distinctive graphic pattern based on the sequence of depolarization and repolarization through the atria and the ventricles. Depolarization refers to the process by which the resting potential of a polarized cell becomes less negative. Repolarization, in turn, refers to the process by which a depolarized cell returns to its resting state. (See *Reviewing the electrical basis of the ECG*, page 31.)

To perform cardiac monitoring, you'll apply electrodes to the patient's chest. The electrodes sense the heart's electrical activity and relay the information to a cardiac monitor (an oscilloscope), where the impulses appear as a continuous ECG waveform.

MONITOR FEATURES

Besides providing a visual display of the patient's heart rate and rhythm, most monitors produce a printed record, known as a rhythm strip. By analyzing the rhythm strip, you can evaluate conduction patterns, estimate heart size, assess heart muscle function and size, and recognize abnormalities in electrolyte balances.

Another common monitor feature is an alarm that signals when the heart rate rises above or falls below set limits. Some monitors also recognize and count abnormal beats and activate an alarm when abnormalities occur. Cardiac monitors may have one or more channels, allowing them to survey cardiac activity in one or more patients.

MONITOR TERMINOLOGY

Operating a cardiac monitor isn't difficult once you learn the technique and become familiar with the following terms:
• *artifact*—incidental, extraneous electrical activity apparent on the ECG tracing and typically caused by electrical interference
• *electrodes*—adhesive pads that detect the heart's electrical activity
• *gain*—adjustment of the monitor's ability to sense the amplitude (size) of the QRS complex
• *ground*—ECG lead that prevents electrical interference ("noise") from entering the monitoring circuit
• *lead*—both the actual color-coded wire that connects the electrode to the monitor cable and the placement of the wire and electrode, which provides different views of the heart's electrical activity. Each lead consists of a positive pole and a negative pole that sense the amplitude and direction of electrical current within the heart. Standard ECG leads reflect 12 views of cardiac activity and are known as leads I, II, III, aV_R, aV_L, aV_F, V_1, V_2, V_3, V_4, V_5, and V_6.

Marilyn Sawyer Sommers, RN, PhD, CCRN, who contributed to this section, is an assistant professor in the College of Nursing and Health at the University of Cincinnati. The publisher also thanks *Hill-Rom,* Batesville, Ind., and *Hewlett-Packard Co.,* Waltham, Mass., for their help.

Understanding the ECG grid

To decipher your patient's electrocardiogram (ECG), begin with the paper it's printed on. Composed of parallel horizontal and vertical lines that form a grid, ECG paper allows you to measure time and amplitude. You need to know these two values to identify certain cardiac irregularities and the patient's heart rate.

To understand the grid, place a strip of ECG graph paper in front of you. Look at the configuration of the squares. Notice how the darker horizontal and vertical lines define large square boxes containing 25 small squares.

Measuring time

The ECG machine traces electrical activity onto the ECG paper at a standard speed of 25 mm/second. Each small square on the horizontal plane represents 0.04 second. Similarly, five small squares represent 0.2 second, and five large squares measure 1 second. You'll use these squares to compute the PR interval and the duration of the QRS complex.

Measuring amplitude

The ECG paper's vertical plane quantifies the amplitude of cardiac electrical activity. Each vertical line falls 1 mm from the next vertical line, with each small square measuring 1 mm × 1 mm. These squares join to form the height and width of a large box. On the vertical plane, these blocks measure the magnitude (or voltage) of a QRS complex, for example. Typically, a 1-millivolt (mV) electrical charge produces a 10-mm deflection on the ECG grid.

Applying the information

Printed along the upper edge of the ECG paper are regularly spaced, short vertical lines denoting additional intervals. With the ECG machine set at standard paper speed, the distance between two consecutive short vertical lines is 75 mm, or 3 seconds, and between every third short vertical line 150 mm, or 6 seconds. By counting the cardiac cycles in one 6-second interval and then multiplying that sum by 10, you'll learn the patient's heart rate.

ECG graph paper

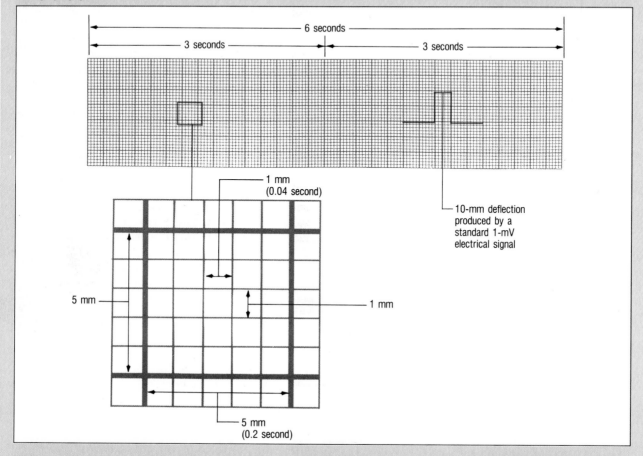

INSIGHTS AND INTERPRETATIONS

Reviewing the electrical basis of the ECG

The graphic waves on your patient's electrocardiogram (ECG) show the direction and magnitude of electrical current, which is generated by atrial and ventricular depolarization and repolarization. Each part of the ECG shows a different phase of cardiac activity.

As shown here, the P wave represents atrial depolarization. The Ta wave—obscured by the QRS complex—represents atrial repolarization, which occurs at the same time as ventricular depolarization (reflected in the QRS complex). The T wave represents ventricular repolarization.

Other factors affecting the ECG waveform include the adequacy of cardiac perfusion and the heart's ability to initiate and conduct the electrical impulse.

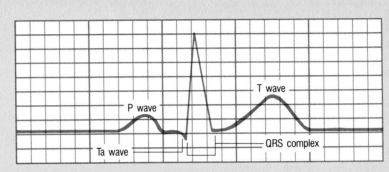

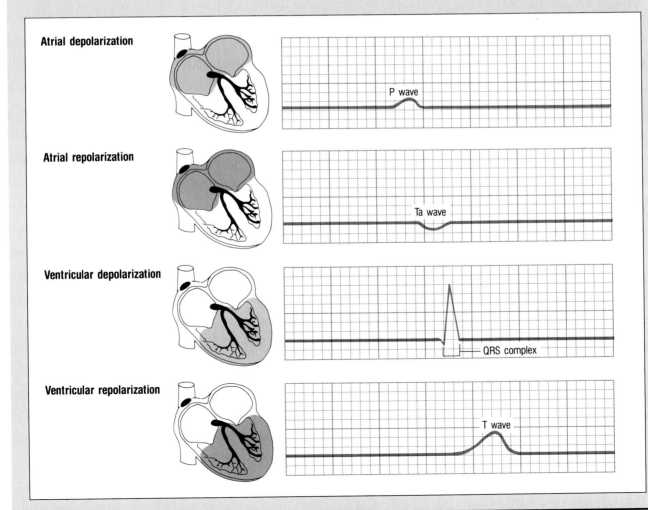

PERFORMING HARDWIRE MONITORING

With hardwire monitoring, your patient and the cardiac monitor are connected by electrodes, leadwires, and a cable. Most hardwire monitors are mounted permanently on a shelf or a wall near the patient's bed. However, some may be mounted on an I.V. pole (for portability), and some may include defibrillators.

The monitor continuously displays the patient's cardiac rhythm and transmits the electrocardiogram (ECG) tracing to a console at a main control station on the nursing unit. Used most commonly in critical care units and emergency departments, hardwire monitoring allows continuous observation of one or more patients from more than one area in the unit.

FEATURES

To track cardiac activity, most hardwire monitors include a three-electrode system, consisting of a positive lead, a negative lead, and a ground lead.

By repositioning these leads, you can detect electrical activity in different areas of the patient's heart. Less prevalent but even more precise are other hardwire systems that use four or five leads. These systems allow you to assess cardiac activity in various areas of the heart without repositioning the electrodes. (See *Comparing lead placement systems.*)

Besides monitoring cardiac rhythm, most monitors available today can track other critical functions, such as pulmonary artery pressure, arterial blood pressure and central venous pressure, cardiac output, body temperature, respiratory rate, and oxygen saturation. Some monitors extend these capabilities to include the analysis of ST segments and the measurement of carbon dioxide pressure in the patient's airway.

Of the available hardwire monitoring systems, some are easier to use than others. For example, adjustments and selections on Siemens and SpaceLabs systems can be made by touching the monitor screen rather than by manipulating knobs and buttons.

Comparing lead placement systems

For most cardiac monitoring, you'll use a three-electrode system. But to increase monitoring capability, you may use a four- or five-electrode system.

Three-electrode system
This system has one positive electrode, one negative electrode, and a ground. Typically, you'll place these electrodes in lead II position, although sometimes you'll use modified chest lead (MCL) placements—specifically MCL_1 or MCL_6. The following describes the differences in leads:
• Lead II records the electrical potential difference between the right arm (negative lead) and the left leg (positive lead). This lead produces clear QRS complexes (which reflect ventricular activity) and positive P waves (showing atrial activity).
• MCL_1 records the sequence of ventricular depolarization more clearly than the other leads, making this

lead a better choice for differentiating between right or left bundle-branch block and ectopy.
• MCL_6, another modified chest lead, clearly visualizes tall QRS complexes, making this the lead of choice for identifying right bundle-branch block, ST-segment abnormalities, and T-wave changes.

Four- and five-electrode systems
In a four-electrode system, a right leg electrode becomes a permanent ground for all leads. In a five-electrode system, an additional exploratory chest lead allows you to monitor any of six modified chest leads as well as the standard limb leads.

Preparing the equipment and the patient

To evaluate your patient's ECG with hardwire monitoring, you'll need a cardiac monitor. You'll also need a monitor cable, leadwires, electrodes, a dry washcloth or gauze pad, alcohol sponges, and the patient's medical record.

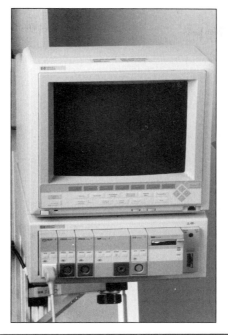
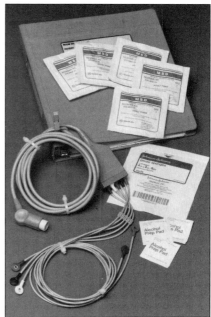

Plug in the monitor and switch on the power. If the cable isn't already connected to the monitor, attach it now.

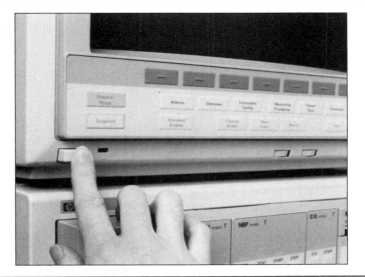

Connect the leadwires to the correct positions on the cable (as shown). If you must connect individual leadwires to the cable and the wires and cable are color-coded, make sure that the color on the leadwire matches the color on the cable. If they're not color-coded, check carefully to make sure that you attach the right arm (RA) wire to the RA outlet on the cable, the left arm (LA) wire to the LA outlet, and so on.

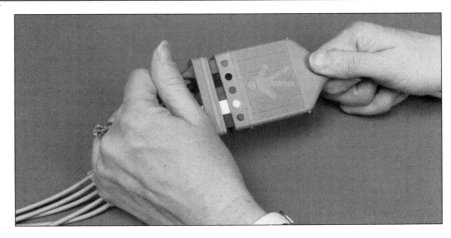

Open the package of electrodes, and attach an electrode to the end of each leadwire.

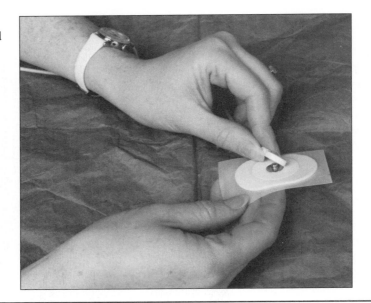

Wash your hands. Explain the procedure to the patient and provide privacy. Expose the patient's chest, and select the electrode sites for the chosen lead arrangement. Then, using a special rough patch on the electrode, a dry washcloth, or a gauze pad, briskly rub each site (as shown) until it reddens. Be sure not to damage or break the skin. Rubbing the skin promotes better electrical contact because this removes dead skin cells. If the patient has an extremely hairy chest, shave about 4″ (10 cm) of hair from each site. Dry these areas.

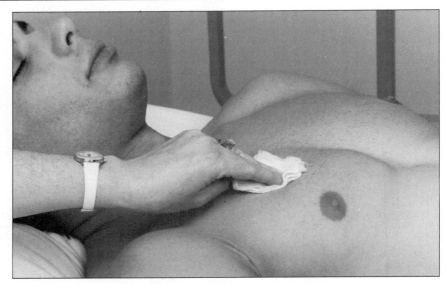

If the patient has oily skin, clean each site with an alcohol sponge. Let the areas dry completely to ensure proper adhesion and to prevent alcohol from becoming trapped underneath the electrode, which could irritate the skin and cause breakdown.

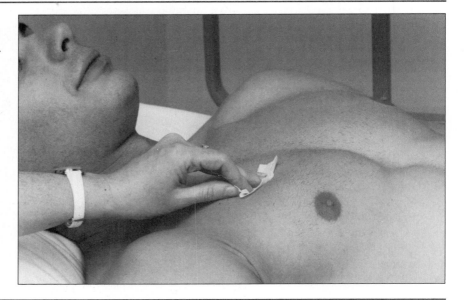

Remove the backing from the pre-gelled electrode. Check the gel. It should be moist. If it's dry, discard the electrode and obtain another one.

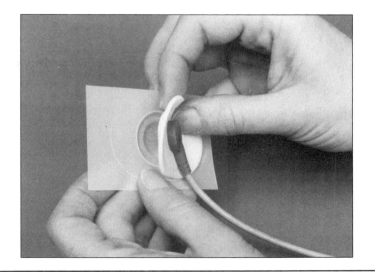

Apply one electrode to each site. To do so, press one side of the electrode against the patient's skin, pull gently, and then press the opposite side of the electrode against the skin. Then use two fingers (as shown) to press on the electrode in a circular pattern. This fixes the gel and stabilizes the electrode. Repeat this process for each electrode.

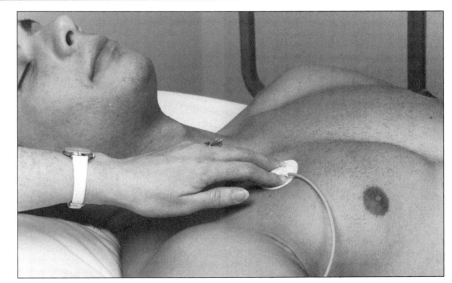

Placing the electrodes

To monitor leads I, II, and III with a three-electrode system, place the color-coded electrodes in the following areas: white electrode just below the right clavicle, black electrode just below the left clavicle, and red electrode on the lower left anterior rib cage. Then turn the lead selector on the monitor to the desired setting (lead I, II, or III). *Note:* The photos use these abbreviations: RA, right arm; LA, left arm; RL, right leg; LL, left leg; and C, chest.

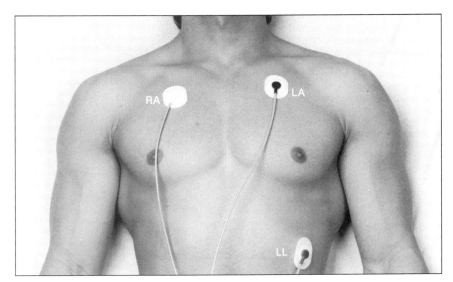

To monitor modified chest lead I (MCL$_1$) with a three-electrode system, turn the lead selector on the monitor to MCL$_1$. If the monitor doesn't have an MCL$_1$ selection, turn the selector to lead III. Then place the white electrode just below the right clavicle, the black electrode just below the left clavicle, and the red electrode over the fourth intercostal space at the right sternal border.

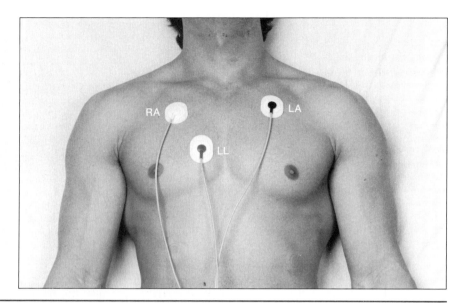

To monitor MCL$_6$ with a three-electrode system, turn the lead selector to MCL$_6$. If the monitor doesn't have an MCL$_6$ selection, turn the selector to lead III. Then place the white electrode just below the right clavicle, the black electrode just below the left clavicle, and the red electrode over the fifth intercostal space at the left midaxillary line.

▶ *Clinical tip:* When placing electrodes, select sites over soft tissue or close to bone. Avoid placing electrodes over muscle, bony prominences, or skin folds because these placements may produce waveform artifacts.

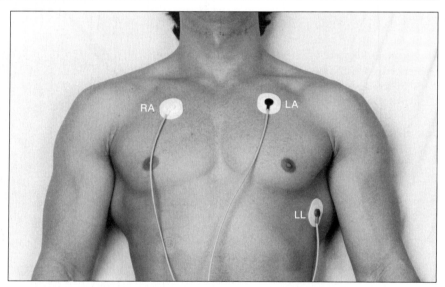

You can monitor any of the 12 standard leads, MCL$_1$, or MCL$_6$ with a five-electrode system. To monitor common leads I, II, III, and MCL$_1$, turn the lead selector on the monitor to the appropriate lead. Then place the white electrode just below the right clavicle, the black electrode just below the left clavicle, the green electrode on the right lower anterior rib cage, the red electrode on the left lower anterior rib cage, and the brown electrode over the fourth intercostal space at the right sternal border (the V$_1$ position).

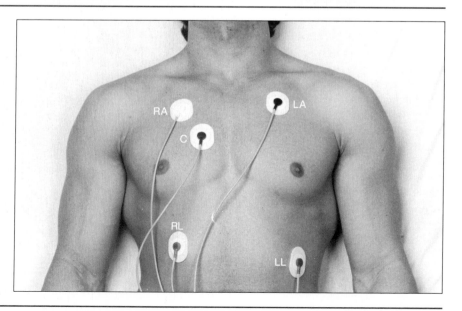

To monitor MCL$_6$ with a five-electrode system, turn the lead selector to MCL$_6$. If the monitor doesn't have an MCL$_6$ selection, turn the selector to lead III. Then place the white electrode just below the right clavicle, the black electrode just below the left clavicle, the green electrode on the right lower anterior rib cage, the red electrode on the left lower anterior rib cage, and the brown electrode over the fifth intercostal space at the left midaxillary line.

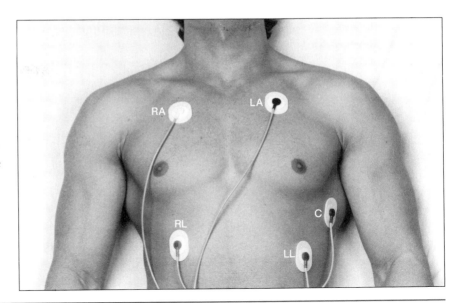

Adjusting the monitor and obtaining a rhythm strip

After you've applied all of the electrodes, observe the monitor screen. You should see the patient's ECG waveform. Assess the quality of the waveform. If the size of the tracing is too large or too small, change the size by adjusting the gain control. If the waveform appears too high or too low on the monitor screen, use the position dial to adjust the position.

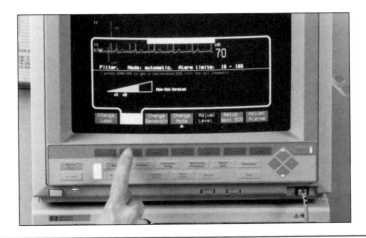

Verify that the monitor detects each heartbeat by taking the patient's apical pulse and comparing it with the digital heart rate display.

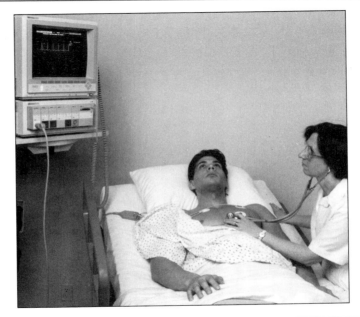

Set the upper and lower limits of the heart rate alarm on the cardiac monitor according to your hospital's policy.

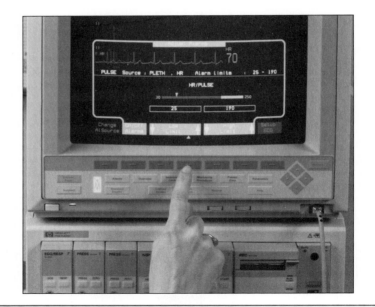

To obtain a printout of the patient's cardiac rhythm, press the RECORD control on the monitor.

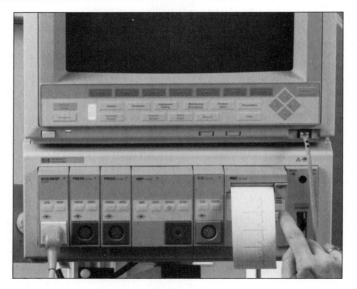

Label the rhythm strip with the patient's name, room number, date, time, and rhythm interpretation. Place the rhythm strip in the appropriate section of the patient's medical record.

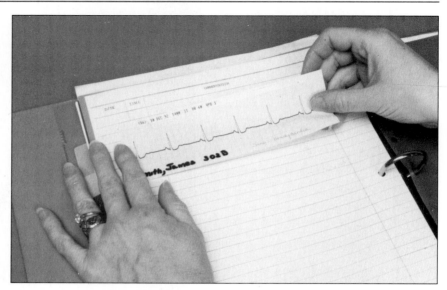

INSIGHTS AND INTERPRETATIONS

Reading rhythm strips

To help you quickly and accurately read your patient's rhythm strip, follow these steps:
• Identify the QRS complexes (which represent ventricular depolarization), and decide whether the patient's ventricular rhythm is regular or irregular.
• Count the QRS complexes within a certain interval to compute the patient's ventricular rate.
• Identify the P waves (which represent atrial depolarization) and determine whether each one precedes a QRS complex.
• Count the number of P waves within a certain time span to determine the atrial rate.
• Analyze the P wave's shape to assess atrial contraction.
• Identify the pacemaker site (the heartbeat's source).
• Measure the PR interval, the QRS complex, and the QT interval.
• Analyze the T wave's shape.
• Identify the rhythm.

To further help you interpret your patient's rhythm strip, review the ECG strips on this page. The first shows normal sinus rhythm; the rest show common arrhythmias.

Normal sinus rhythm
Impulses originate in the sinoatrial (SA) node, travel normally through the conduction system, and generate a regular rhythm of 60 to 100 beats/minute.

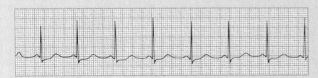

Sinus bradycardia
In this arrhythmia, impulses originate in the SA node but produce fewer than 60 beats/minute.

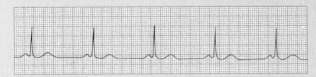

Sinus tachycardia
In this arrhythmia, impulses originate in the SA node and produce a regular rhythm of more than 100 beats/minute.

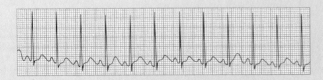

Atrial flutter
In this rhythm strip, note the rapid atrial rate, which produces 260 to 360 flutter waves/minute. The atrial rhythm is regular, but the P waves have a saw-toothed appearance. The ventricular rate is also rapid (about 150 beats/minute).

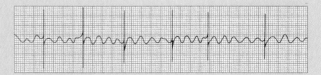

Atrial fibrillation
This rhythm strip shows classic atrial fibrillation. Multiple pacemaker sites produce between 350 and 600 fibrillation waves/minute. These waves have an abnormal, chaotic, and irregular appearance. The ventricular rate is also rapid and can be as high as 200 beats/minute.

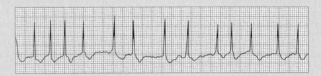

Ventricular tachycardia
In this arrhythmia, three or more premature ventricular contractions occur in succession—the rate ranges from 110 to 250 beats/minute. P waves may or may not appear.

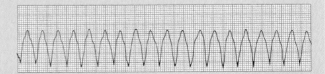

Ventricular fibrillation
On this rhythm strip, note the absence of coordinated ventricular beats. In ventricular fibrillation, the ventricles contract chaotically and irregularly from 300 to 500 times/minute.

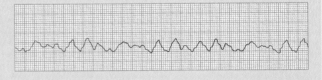

Managing cardiac monitoring problems

PROBLEM	POSSIBLE CAUSES	SOLUTIONS
False-high-rate alarm	• Monitor interpreting large T waves as QRS complexes, which doubles the rate • Skeletal muscle activity	• Reposition electrodes to lead where QRS complexes are taller than the T waves. • Place electrodes away from major muscle masses.
False-low-rate alarm	• Shift in electrical axis caused by patient movement, making QRS complexes too small to register • Low amplitude of QRS complex • Poor contact between electrodes and skin	• Reapply electrodes. Set gain so that height of complex exceeds 1 mV. • Increase gain. • Reapply electrodes.
Low amplitude	• Gain dial set too low • Poor contact between skin and electrodes; dried gel; broken or loose leadwires; poor connection between patient and monitor; malfunctioning monitor; physiologic loss of amplitude of QRS complex	• Increase gain. • Check connections on all leadwires and monitoring cable. Replace or reapply electrodes as necessary.
Wandering baseline	• Poor electrode placement or contact with skin • Thoracic movement with respirations	• Reposition or replace electrodes. • Reposition electrodes.
Artifact (waveform interference)	• Patient having seizures, chills, or anxiety • Patient movement • Electrodes applied improperly • Static electricity • Electrical short circuit in leadwires or cable • Interference from decreased room humidity	• Notify doctor and treat patient as ordered. Keep patient warm and reassure him. • Help patient relax. • Check electrodes and reapply, if necessary. • Make sure cables don't have exposed connectors. Change static-causing bedclothes. • Replace broken equipment. Use stress loops when applying leadwires. • Regulate humidity to 40%.
Broken leadwires or cable	• Tension on leadwires due to repeated pulling • Cables and leadwires cleaned with alcohol or acetone, causing brittleness	• Replace leadwires and retape them, making sure to tape part of the wire into a loop. This absorbs tension that would otherwise tug at the ends of the wire. • Clean cable and leadwires with soapy water. *Do not let cable ends get wet.* Replace cable as necessary.
60-cycle interference (fuzzy baseline)	• Electrical interference from other equipment in room • Patient's bed improperly grounded	• Attach all electrical equipment to common ground. Check plugs to make sure prongs aren't loose. • Attach bed ground to the room's common ground.
Skin excoriation under electrode	• Patient allergic to electrode adhesive • Electrode remaining on skin too long	• Remove electrodes and apply nonallergenic electrodes and nonallergenic tape. • Remove electrode, clean site, and reapply electrode at new site.

PERFORMING TELEMETRY MONITORING

Battery powered and portable, telemetry provides continuous electrocardiogram (ECG) monitoring without attaching the patient directly to a hardwire monitoring system. Telemetry frees the patient from cumbersome wires and cables. This system also allows him to be comfortably mobile and safely isolated from the electrical leakage and accidental shock occasionally associated with hardwire monitoring.

Telemetry is especially useful for monitoring arrhythmias that occur during sleep, rest, exercise, or stressful situations. Unlike hardwire monitoring, telemetry can monitor only cardiac rate and rhythm.

Preparing the equipment and the patient

For telemetry, the patient wears from two to five electrodes. Aided by a small transmitter that the patient carries in a pocket or a pouch, the electrodes detect and transmit the heart's electrical activity. The transmitter sends signals to an antenna that relays the impulses to a monitor at a nursing station.

To institute telemetry monitoring, obtain a transmitter, a transmitter pouch, a telemetry battery pack, leads, and electrodes.

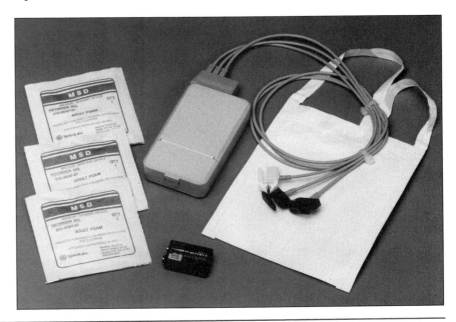

Insert a new battery into the transmitter. Be sure to match the poles on the battery with the polar markings on the transmitter case.

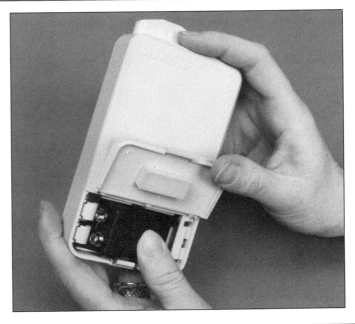

By pressing the button at the top of the unit (as shown), test the battery's charge and test the unit to ensure that the battery is operational.

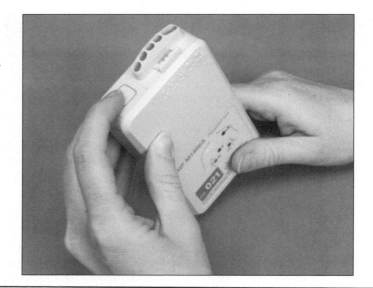

If the leadwires aren't permanently affixed to the telemetry unit, attach them securely. If leadwires must be attached individually, be sure to connect each one to the correct outlet.

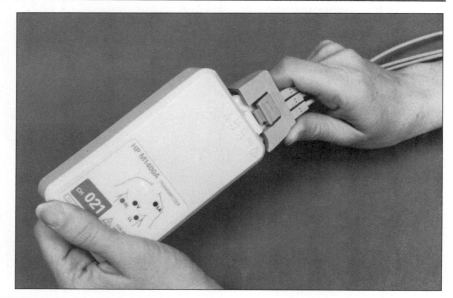

Wash your hands. Explain the procedure to the patient and provide privacy. Expose the patient's chest, and select the lead arrangement. Remove the backing from one of the gelled electrodes. Check the gel for moisture. If it's dry, discard the electrode and obtain a new one.

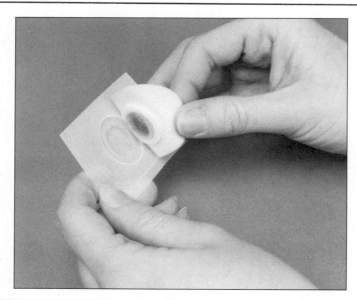

Apply the electrode to the appropriate site by pressing one side of the electrode against the patient's skin, pulling gently, and then pressing the other side against the skin. Press your fingers in a circular motion around the electrode to fix the gel and stabilize the electrode. Repeat for each electrode.

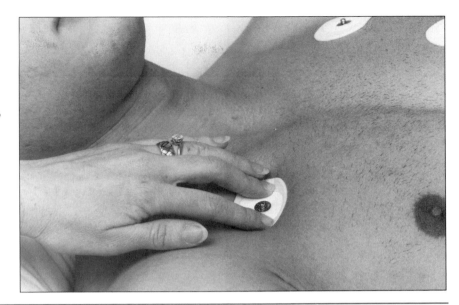

Attach an electrode to the end of each leadwire.

▷ **Clinical tip:** If you're using a clip-type electrode (as shown), attach the leadwire to the electrode after the electrode is in place on the chest. If you're using a snap-type leadwire, attach the leadwire to the electrode before you put the electrode on the chest.

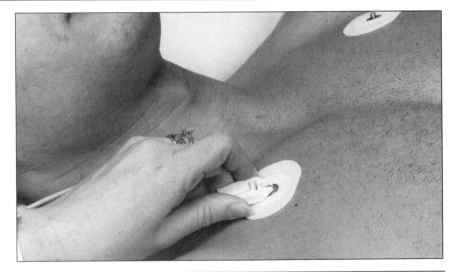

Place the transmitter in the pouch. Tie the pouch strings around the patient's neck and waist. Make sure that the pouch fits snugly without causing the patient discomfort. If no pouch is available, place the transmitter in the patient's bathrobe pocket.

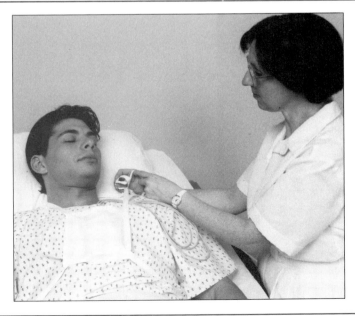

Check with the telemetry central station to ensure that the waveform transmits properly. If necessary, ask the patient to remain resting or sitting in his room while you locate his telemetry monitor at the central station. Evaluate the waveform for clarity, position, and size. Adjust the gain and baseline as needed.

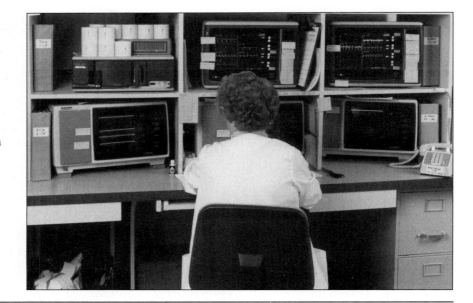

To obtain a rhythm strip, press the RECORD key at the central station. Label the rhythm strip with the patient's name, room number, date, and time. Also identify the rhythm. Place the rhythm strip in the appropriate location in the patient's chart. Document the interpretation of the rhythm on the patient record.

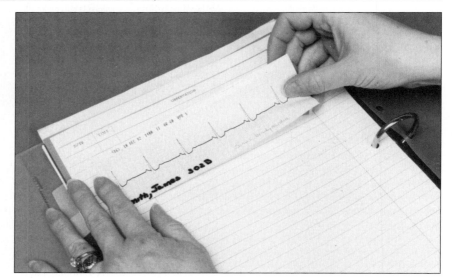

Teaching telemetry patients

To promote cooperation during telemetry monitoring, explain the procedure to the patient and allow him to ask questions. Use the following instructions as a guide.

• Show the patient the transmitter unit and explain how it works.
• Inform him that the unit won't produce sufficient electrical current to cause a shock.
• If applicable, show him the button on the transmitter that will produce a recording of his electrocardiogram at the central station. Teach him how to push the button whenever he experiences chest pain, palpitations, or related symptoms.

• Instruct the patient to remove the transmitter unit before taking a bath or shower. Stress, however, that he needs to let you know before he removes the unit.
• Explain that the telemetry unit can transmit signals only a set distance from the central station. Let the patient know how far he can move from the central station before the transmission will be interrupted.

PERFORMING 12-LEAD ELECTROCARDIOGRAPHY

A valuable diagnostic tool, 12-lead electrocardiography (ECG) graphically records the heart's electrical activity. In this procedure, electrical impulses created by the heart's conduction system can be monitored by electrodes attached to the skin. These electrodes sense the electric currents and transmit them to an instrument that produces a record of cardiac activity. The printed record, or waveform, is the electrocardiogram.

UNDERSTANDING LEADS

To assess cardiac activity using a standard 12-lead ECG, you'll position a series of electrodes on the patient's extremities and chest wall. The 12 leads include three bipolar limb leads (I, II, and III), three unipolar augmented limb leads (aV_R, aV_L, and aV_F), and six unipolar precordial, or chest, leads (V_1, V_2, V_3, V_4, V_5, and V_6). By recording data from 12 different leads, or perspectives, this type of ECG provides a composite picture of the heart's electrical activity. Because each lead displays cardiac electrical activity from a different perspective, the waveform resulting from a particular lead will have its own characteristic pattern.

Limb leads

The six limb leads reflect electrical activity in the heart's frontal plane. In this plane—a vertical view through the middle of the heart from top to bottom—electrical activity is recorded from the anterior to the posterior axis.

Leads I, II, and III are called bipolar because they require two electrodes—one positive and one negative. These leads record the potential difference (the work required to transport an electric charge from one point to another) between the two electrodes. Lead I records the potential difference between the right arm and the left arm. Lead II records the potential difference between the right arm and the left leg. Lead III records the potential difference between the left arm and the left leg. (See *Einthoven's triangle,* page 46.)

Augmented limb leads aV_R, aV_L, and aV_F are called unipolar because they have only one electrode—the positive pole. The negative pole is computed by the ECG machine. Without augmentation,

the tracings from these leads would be quite small. The ECG machine automatically enlarges (or augments) the deflections to make them more readable. When the positive pole is the right arm, the lead is known as the aV_R (augmented vector right) lead; when the positive pole is the left arm, the lead is known as the aV_L (augmented vector left) lead; when the positive pole is the left leg, the lead is known as the aV_F (augmented vector foot) lead.

Chest leads

The six unipolar precordial leads provide information on electrical activity in the heart's horizontal plane—a transverse view through the middle of the heart, dividing it into upper and lower portions. In this plane, electrical activity can be seen from a superior or an inferior approach.

These leads are placed at six sites over the anterior surface of the chest and connected to the positive terminal of the ECG machine. The negative electrode, called the indifferent electrode, is connected to the arms and left leg at the same time.

Leads V_1 and V_2 monitor the right side of the heart, so they're often referred to as the right precordial leads. In contrast, leads V_3 through V_6 are called the left precordial leads because they monitor the heart's left side.

By reviewing the ECG tracings from all the leads, you'll obtain a fairly complete view of the electrical activity in the heart's inferior, anterior, and lateral portions. The leads are grouped together and called inferior leads, anterior leads, or lateral leads based on the area they scan. The inferior leads are leads II, III, and aV_F; the anterior leads, leads V_1, V_2, V_3 and V_4; and the lateral leads, leads I, aV_L, V_5, and V_6. Lead aV_R doesn't provide a specific view of the heart but does reflect changes in electrical activity.

OPERATING THE RECORDER

The ECG machine can be a multichannel or a single-channel recorder. For a multichannel recording, you'll attach all electrodes to the patient at once, and the machine will print a simultaneous view of all leads. For a single-channel recording, you'll systematically attach and remove selected electrodes, stopping and starting the tracing each time.

Contributors to this section include *Marilyn Sawyer Sommers, RN, PhD, CCRN,* an assistant professor at the University of Cincinnati College of Nursing and Health Sciences, and *Paulette Dorney, RN, MSN, CCRN,* an instructor in the Department of Critical Care Staff Development at North Penn Hospital, Lansdale, Pa. The publisher thanks *Doylestown (Pa.) Hospital* and *Hewlett-Packard Co.,* Waltham, Mass., for their help.

Einthoven's triangle

The axes of the three bipolar limb leads (I, II, and III) form a triangle, known as Einthoven's triangle, that is the model for the standard limb leads in electrocardiography. Because the electrodes for these leads are placed about equidistant from the heart, the triangle is equilateral.

The axis of lead I extends from shoulder to shoulder, with the right arm lead being the negative electrode and the left arm lead being the positive electrode. The axis of lead II runs from the negative right arm lead electrode to the positive left leg lead electrode. The axis of lead III extends from the negative left arm lead electrode to the positive left leg lead electrode.

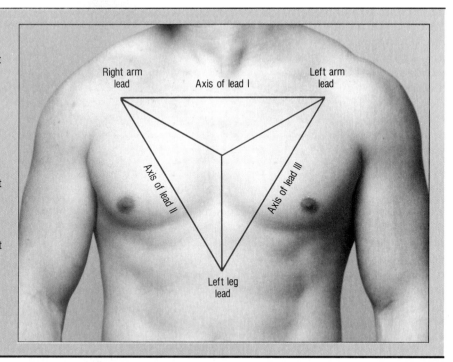

Using a multichannel ECG machine

Begin by gathering the necessary equipment. You'll need a multichannel ECG machine, such as the one shown at right. You'll also need recording paper, pregelled disposable electrodes (or reusable electrodes with suction bulbs and rubber straps and electrode paste or gel), and 4" × 4" gauze pads or a moist cloth towel. Optional equipment includes a drape, shaving supplies, and a marking pen.

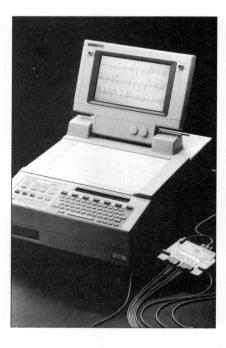

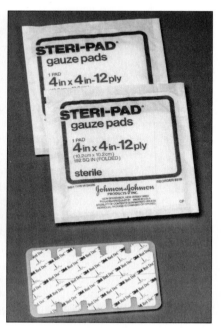

Inform the patient that his doctor has ordered an ECG and explain the procedure. Tell the patient that the procedure will take about 10 minutes and that it's a safe and painless way to evaluate cardiac function. Set up the equipment at the patient's bedside.

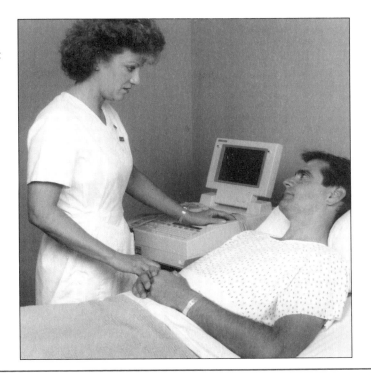

Plug the cord into a grounded outlet, and place the patient in a supine position. If he can't tolerate lying flat, help him to semi-Fowler's position. Uncover his chest, and expose his arms and legs. Always maintain his privacy.

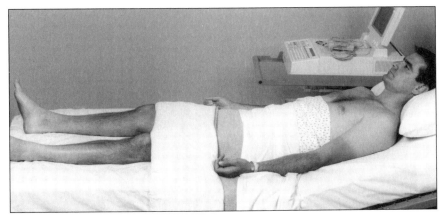

Attach the limb leads to hair-free sites on the arms and legs. A flat, fleshy site is best; try to avoid bony or muscular areas. The inner aspect of the wrist and the inner aspect of the ankle are usually good contact sites. Clean each site to remove skin oil and to increase contact with the electrodes, following the electrode manufacturer's guidelines for skin preparation.

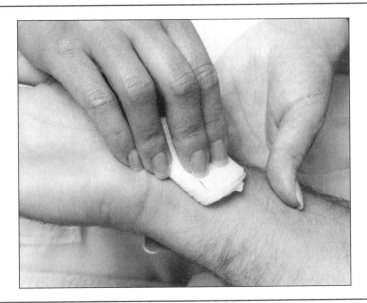

Apply electrode paste or gel, or the disposable electrodes (as shown), to the inner aspects of the wrists and the medial aspects of the ankles. If you're using paste or gel, rub it into the skin. If you're using disposable electrodes, peel off the contact paper and apply them to the site. Position leg electrodes with the lead connections pointing up.

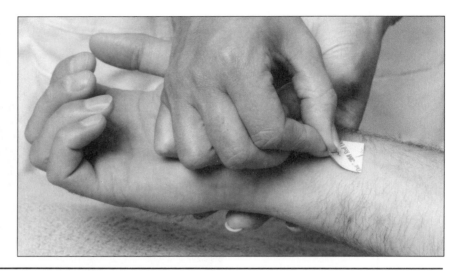

Connect the limb leadwires to the electrodes. Make sure that metal parts are clean to ensure a good electrical connection.

▶ **Clinical tip:** The tip of each leadwire is lettered and color coded for easy identification. The white (or RA) leadwire goes to the right arm; the green (or RL) leadwire, to the right leg; the red (or LL) leadwire, to the left leg; the black (or LA) leadwire, to the left arm; and the brown (or V_1 to V_6) leadwires, to the chest.

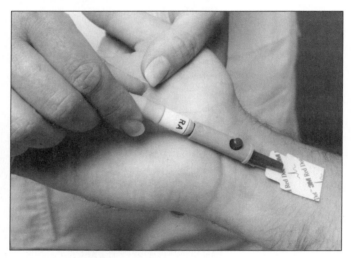

Prepare the anterior chest sites as you did the extremities. Attach the chest leads to the six anterior chest sites (as shown). If the patient is a woman, place the chest electrodes below the breast tissue.

Make sure that all leads are securely attached; then turn on the machine. Tell the patient to relax, lie still, and breathe normally. Advise him not to talk when you record his ECG because muscle movement may distort the ECG tracing.

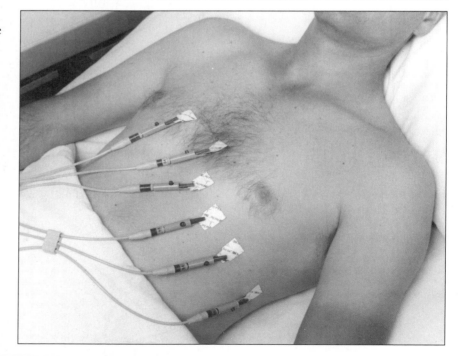

Make sure that the ECG paper speed selector is set to the standard 25 mm/second. Then, if necessary, enter the appropriate patient identification data. Calibrate or standardize the machine according to the manufacturer's recommendation. The machine will record a normal standardization mark—a square that's the height of 2 large squares or 10 small squares on the recording paper.

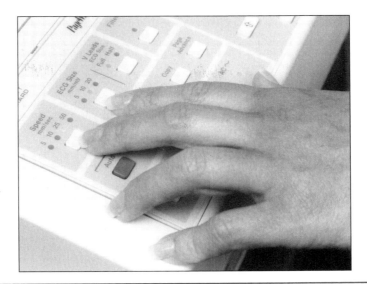

Press the AUTO button and record the ECG. Observe the tracing quality. The machine will record all 12 leads automatically, recording three consecutive leads simultaneously. When the machine finishes recording the 12-lead ECG, turn it off. Remove the electrodes and clean the patient's skin. Use a moist cloth towel or a 4″ × 4″ gauze pad to remove any residual paste or gel from the patient's skin.

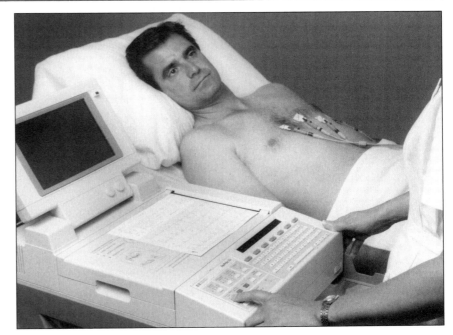

Help the patient into his gown and cover him. Raise the head of the bed, and assist him to a comfortable position. Then document the procedure. Note any changes in his condition, such as chest pain or shortness of breath. Also note any unusual electrode placements—necessitated by a dressing in place or an I.V. line, for example. Write his name and room number, the date and time, and his doctor's name on the ECG strip, and place the strip in his chart.

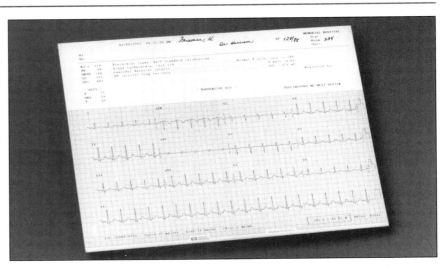

Using a single-channel ECG machine

Before you begin, obtain the single-channel ECG machine, recording paper, pregelled disposable electrodes (or reusable electrodes with rubber straps [with or without suction bulbs] and electrode paste or gel), and 4" × 4" gauze pads (or skin preparation pads). Optional equipment includes a drape, shaving supplies, a marking pen, and a moist cloth towel.

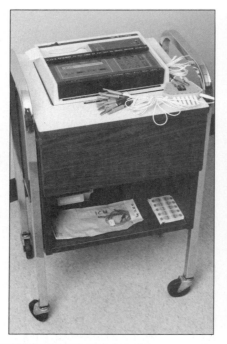 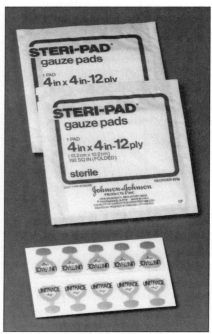

Explain the procedure to the patient, and assemble the equipment at his bedside. Place him in a supine position. If necessary for comfort, elevate the head of the bed slightly. Then uncover his arms and legs, and drape him appropriately. Always maintain his privacy.

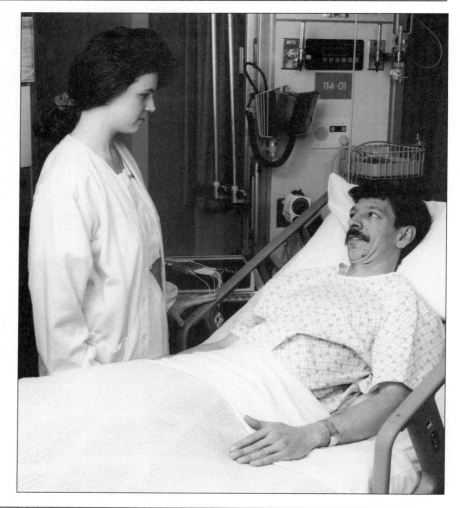

Select sites for limb lead attachment that are flat, fleshy, and hair-free; avoid bony and muscular areas. The inner aspects of the wrists and the medial aspects of the ankles are good choices. Following the manufacturer's guidelines for skin preparation, clean the sites to remove skin oil and improve electrode contact.

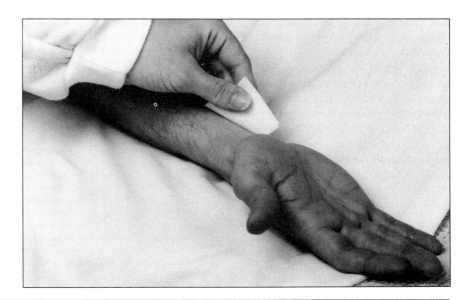

Apply the disposable electrodes to each of the four limbs. (If you're using reusable electrodes, apply the electrode paste or gel to each electrode before applying it to the skin.)

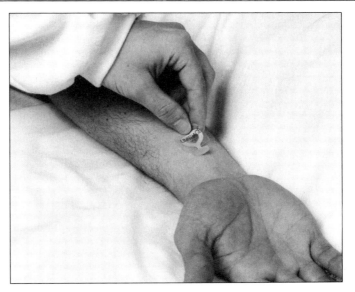

Clip each limb leadwire to the limb electrodes, matching each limb leadwire to the corresponding electrode. Each leadwire is color coded (and possibly letter coded) as follows: white (RA) for right arm, green (RL) for right leg, red (LL) for left leg, and black (LA) for left arm.

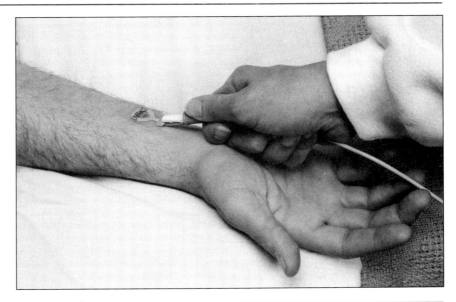

Alternatively, if you have reusable electrodes, place the metal electrodes on top of the paste or gel.

▶ *Clinical tip:* If you're using paste or gel, secure the electrode promptly after applying the conductive medium to prevent it from drying before use. Never substitute alcohol or acetone pads for the electrode paste or gel because these pads impair electrode contact with the skin and thus transmission of electrical impulses. Secure the electrode with a rubber strap. Avoid pulling the rubber strap too tightly; this could cause muscle spasms that would distort the ECG tracings. Then connect the limb leadwires to the electrodes (as shown).

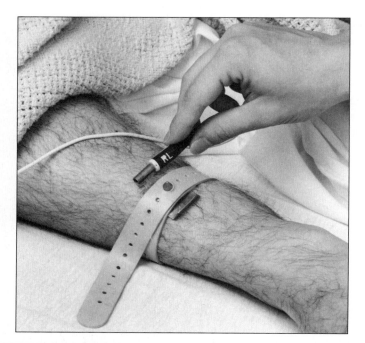

After connecting the machine to its power source, turn it on by pressing the ON-OFF switch. Then standardize or calibrate the machine according to the manufacturer's instructions. Watch for the standardization marks to appear on the ECG tracing (as shown).

▶ *Clinical tip:* To provide a consistent frame of reference throughout the procedure, standardize the machine after you run each lead. Some machines do this automatically.

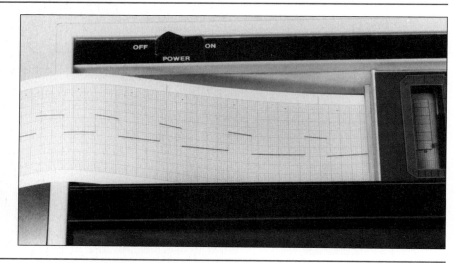

Now you're ready to run the first six leads: I, II, III, aV_R, aV_L, and aV_F. To begin, press the lead I button and run a 6-second strip. Label the strip with the appropriate lead according to your hospital's policy. (*Note:* Some machines, such as the one shown here, automatically mark the strip.)

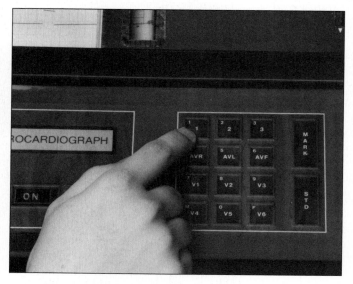

Press each remaining standard limb lead button (leads II and III) and the augmented limb lead buttons (leads aV$_R$, aV$_L$, and aV$_F$), and run a 6-second strip for each lead. Label the strip with the appropriate lead.

▶ *Clinical tip:* If you observe ectopic beats or rhythm changes, run longer strips so that the doctor can observe these irregularities at greater length.

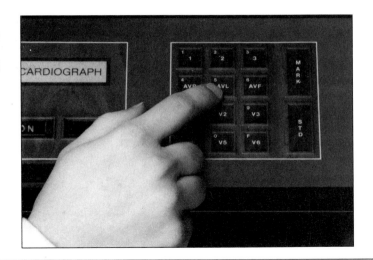

Now expose the patient's chest, being sure to preserve his privacy. Apply the chest leads as indicated at right. If you're using a suction bulb electrode, place the electrode gel or paste at the proper position for lead V$_1$. Then squeeze the rubber bulb of the electrode between your fingers, and place the bulb over the gel. Release your fingers.

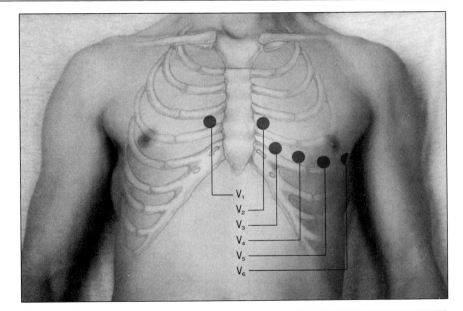

Clip the chest leadwires, which are color coded brown, to the chest electrodes (as shown). Before recording the ECG, make sure that all the leadwires are attached properly and that the electrodes adhere to the chest.

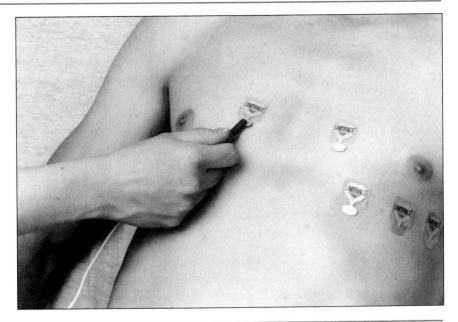

To record cardiac electrical activity from the chest leads, press the V₁ button and run a 6-second strip. Then press the V₂ button and run another 6-second strip. Continue this procedure until you record all six chest leads. (*Note:* If your machine uses a suction bulb electrode, you'll have to reposition this electrode each time you record a lead.)

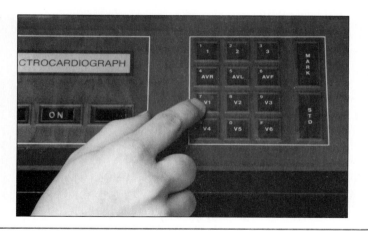

When the ECG is complete, remove the electrodes from the patient's skin. Clean his skin with the moist cloth towel or a *4″ × 4″* gauze pad. Then disconnect the leadwires from the electrodes.

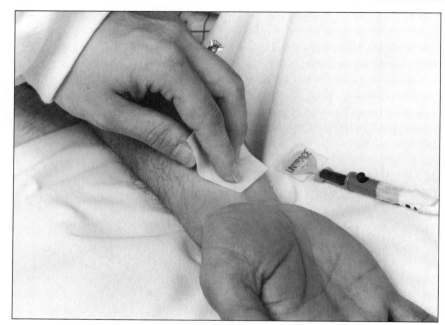

Document the procedure. On the ECG strip, write the patient's name and room number, the date and time, and his doctor's name.

▷ *Clinical tip:* Include any other special information about your patient. For instance, note whether he has an artificial pacemaker or feels any chest pain during the ECG. Also document any unusual electrode placements.

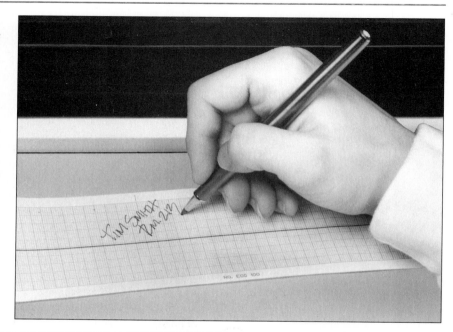

Twelve-lead ECG: A closer look

The 12-lead electrocardiogram (ECG) shows cardiac electrical activity from 12 different directions in relation to the wave of depolarization (shown in color). The waveform from the standard limb leads (I, II, and III) and the three augmented limb leads (aV_R, aV_L, and aV_F) represents the direction of electrical potential throughout the heart (indicated below by arrows). Abnormal waveforms from a particular lead reflect possible damage or dysfunction in that area.

The six precordial leads (V₁, V₂, V₃, V₄, V₅, V₆) represent the direction that electrical potential takes in the ventricles (also shown by directional arrows below at right). Again, waveform abnormalities suggest areas for further investigation.

The chart below lists each lead and the corresponding direction of electrical potential and view of the heart. A normal ECG waveform from that lead also appears.

Keep in mind that a normal ECG waveform has the following characteristics:
• P wave deflection is usually positive but may be diphasic or inverted in leads III, aV₁, and V₁, and may be inverted in aV_R.
• PR intervals are constant in all leads.
• QRS complex deflection changes with the lead, but duration remains constant.
• ST-segment deflection is isoelectric or with minimal deviation.
• T wave deflection should be upright in most leads. This wave is inverted in lead aV_R. Occasionally, deflection is biphasic or inverted in leads III, aV_L, and V₁.

Limb lead vectors

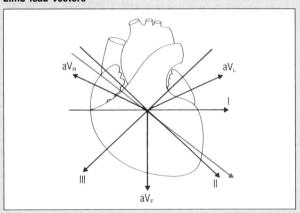

Precordial lead vectors

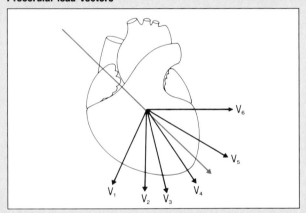

LEAD	DIRECTION OF POTENTIAL	VIEW	NORMAL WAVEFORM
I	Between left arm (positive) and right arm (negative)	Lateral wall	
II	Between left leg (positive) and right arm (negative)	Inferior wall	
III	Between left leg (positive) and left arm (negative)	Inferior wall	

(continued)

Twelve-lead ECG: A closer look *(continued)*

LEAD	DIRECTION OF POTENTIAL	VIEW	NORMAL WAVEFORM
aV_R	Right arm to heart	No specific view	
aV_L	Left arm to heart	Lateral wall	
aV_F	Left leg to heart	Inferior wall	
V_1	Fourth intercostal space, right sternal border, to heart	Anteroseptal wall	
V_2	Fourth intercostal space, left sternal border, to heart	Anteroseptal wall	
V_3	Midway between V_2 and V_4 to heart	Anterior wall	
V_4	Fifth intercostal space, midclavicular line, to heart	Anterior wall	
V_5	Fifth intercostal space, anterior axillary line, to heart	Lateral wall	
V_6	Fifth intercostal space, midaxillary line, to heart	Lateral wall	

PERFORMING SIGNAL-AVERAGED E.C.G.

A simple, noninvasive test, signal-averaged electro-cardiography (ECG) uses a computer to identify late electrical potentials (tiny impulses that follow normal ventricular depolarization). It may help identify patients who have a high risk of sudden death from sustained ventricular tachycardia (VT). Identifying such patients allows the doctor to take preventive measures, such as drug therapy. Test results may also help determine whether the patient is a candidate for invasive procedures, such as electrophysiologic testing or angiography.

Patients who are prone to VT—after myocardial infarction, for example—or those who have unexplained syncope or nonischemic congestive cardiomyopathy typically have late electrical potentials. Although researchers have known about this conduction abnormality for years, they hadn't been able to detect it until the recent development of signal-averaged ECG.

Of course, screening for late potentials isn't foolproof. Some patients with VT may not have late potentials because reentry abnormalities don't always cause this arrhythmia. Or some patients may have late potentials of such low amplitude that the abnormality will be obscured despite signal averaging.

What's more, the test isn't indicated for patients with prolonged QRS complexes (which may conceal late potentials) that result from such conduction abnormalities as bundle-branch blocks, Wolff-Parkinson-White syndrome, or paced ventricular rhythms.

HOW SIGNAL AVERAGING WORKS

The signal-averaged ECG is a noise-free surface ECG recording from three specialized leads for several hundred beats. The computer-assisted tracing results from three processes—amplification, signal averaging, and filtering.

Amplification enlarges late electrical potentials so that they can be recognized. However, it also enlarges other electrical activity or "noises," such as external interference and respiratory and skeletal muscle movement.

At the same time, the computer processes the signals from a series of heartbeats to produce one representative QRS complex without artifacts. Its averaging process cancels out noise that doesn't occur as a repetitious pattern or with the same consistent timing as the QRS complex.

To complete the process, high-pass and low-pass filters reduce additional noise that occurs, for instance, during the ST segment and the T wave. Without this filtering, late electrical potentials would remain hidden. Filtering, however, can't eliminate the noise caused by muscle movement, so you'll need to keep the patient still during the test. (See the patient-teaching aid *Learning about a signal-averaged electrocardiogram,* page 64.) You'll also need to prepare his skin adequately and keep in mind that a slow heart rate and frequent ventricular ectopic beats or aberrant beats may increase the time needed to produce a signal-averaged ECG.

Gather the necessary equipment and take it to the patient's bedside. You'll need a specialized ECG machine (such as the model from Arrhythmia Research Technology at right), electrodes, alcohol sponges, and possibly a razor. You'll also need an IBM-compatible computer to store and print the results.

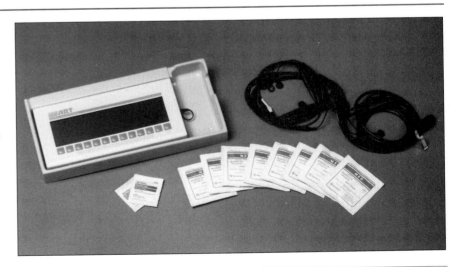

Contributors to this section include *Lynn Lansdowne, RN,C, MSN, CCRN,* Director of Critical Care and Education at Pocono Medical Center, East Stroudsburg, Pa., and *Marylin Schactman, RN, MSN, CCRN,* Assistant Vice-President of Nursing at St. Francis Hospital, Roslyn, N.Y. The publisher thanks *Arrhythmia Research Technology, Inc.,* Austin, Tex., and *Hill-Rom,* Batesville, Ind., for their help.

Explain the procedure to the patient. Tell him that this test records the heart's electrical activity and can identify abnormal rhythms early, when they can be treated. Emphasize that he shouldn't talk or move his head, arms, or body during the procedure. Reassure him that the test takes only about 10 minutes and that no electrical current will enter his body.

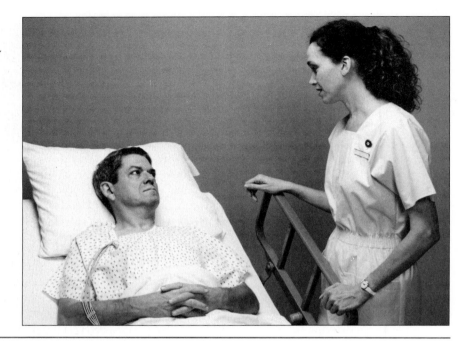

Place the machine close to the patient's bed. If he's connected to a cardiac monitor, remove the monitoring electrodes to accommodate the new electrodes and leadwires and to minimize electrical interference on the signal-averaged tracing. Unplug all unnecessary equipment to decrease extraneous electrical noise.

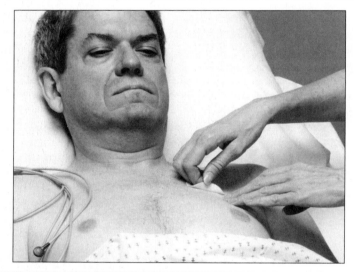

Place the patient in a supine position with his arms at his sides. Drape him appropriately (as shown). Ask him to relax his arms and legs, and keep him warm to minimize shivering or trembling, which can cause electrical interference. Make sure his feet aren't touching the bed's footboard, which can also cause interference.

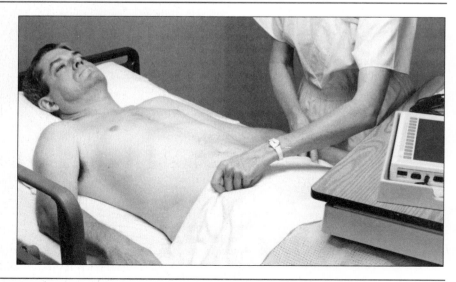

Using an alcohol sponge, prepare the patient's skin for electrode placement (as shown). After the skin dries, lightly scrape it with the edge of the electrode so that the slightly rough surface promotes contact with the electrode.

Avoid applying an electrode to hairy skin. If necessary, shave the area first.

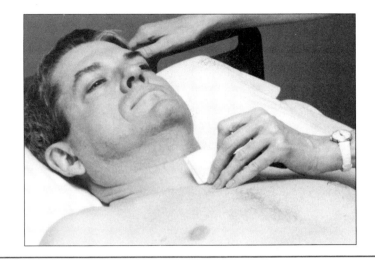

To place electrodes on the patient's chest, select flat, fleshy areas and avoid large muscles or bony prominences. Place the positive X electrode at the left fourth intercostal space, midaxillary line; the negative X electrode at the right fourth intercostal space, midaxillary line; the positive Y electrode at the left iliac crest; the negative Y electrode at the superior aspect of the manubrium of the sternum; the positive Z electrode at the fourth intercostal space, left sternal border (standard V_2 position); and the ground (G) electrode on the lower right at the eighth rib.

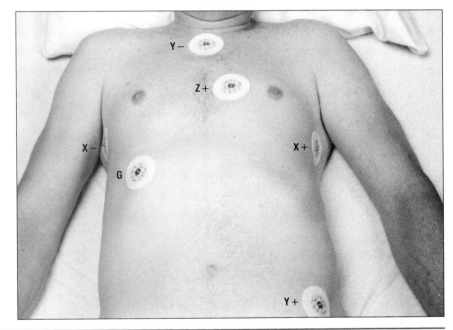

Then have the patient turn over or sit up. Place the negative Z electrode on his back, directly posterior to the positive Z electrode.

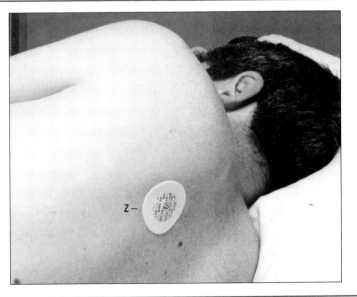

Alternatively, your hospital may use the following electrode placements: the positive X electrode at the left fourth intercostal space, midaxillary line; the negative X electrode at the right fourth intercostal space, midaxillary line; the positive Y electrode at the standard V_3 position; the negative Y electrode at the second intercostal space along the left side of the sternum; the positive Z electrode at the standard V_2 position; and the ground electrode on the lower right side at the eighth rib.

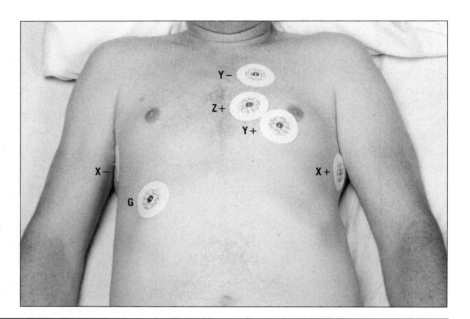

To position the negative Z electrode, have the patient turn over or sit up. Place this electrode on his back, directly posterior to the positive Z electrode. Then help him into a supine position.

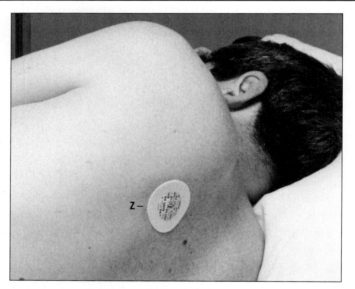

Connect the leadwires to the electrodes. Instruct the patient to lie still with his arms at his sides. Tell him to relax and breathe normally. Also tell him to avoid talking except to inform you if he needs to move, cough, or sneeze. That way, you can stop the recording temporarily.

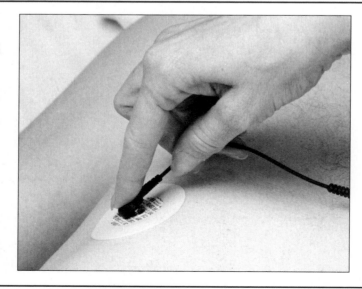

Turn on the machine by pressing the ON/OFF key. Now press the HIR key (as shown) to record a signal-averaged ECG tracing. Check to see that the baseline tracing doesn't show any noise interference. Examine the pattern of the tracing.

Note: To obtain a reliable signal-averaged ECG, check that the patient isn't having ectopic beats.

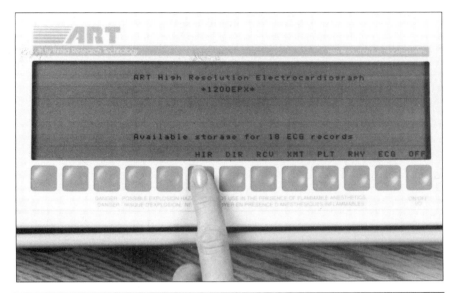

Press the START key. The patient's heart rate will be displayed at the top of the screen. The ECG machine will also store the number of beats recorded and display this number next to the patient's heart rate.

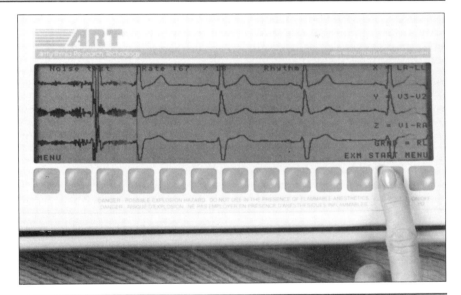

Once you've recorded 50 beats (the monitor will display 50 cycles), press the EXM key to view the current averaged data. Note that once you press the EXM key, the screen will display new codes (as shown).

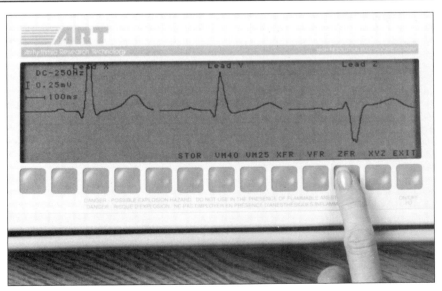

Then press the UM40 key to filter the tracing. Verify that the noise level is 0.3 microvolts (μV) or less and continue recording. Record at least 200 beats.

▶ *Clinical tip:* If the noise level exceeds 0.3 μV, check the electrode connections and make sure that the patient isn't holding onto the bed rails or pressing against the footboard. If you can't decrease the noise level, stop the recording, remove the electrodes, and begin the procedure again.

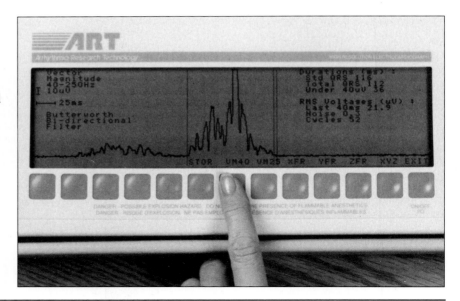

After you've recorded 200 beats with a noise level of 0.3 μV or less, press the STOR key to store the information. Then enter the patient's identifying data into the machine, and turn it off. Remove the electrodes from the patient (as shown) and cover him. Process the information from the signal-averaging apparatus as directed by the operator's manual, and print a tracing for interpretation and documentation.

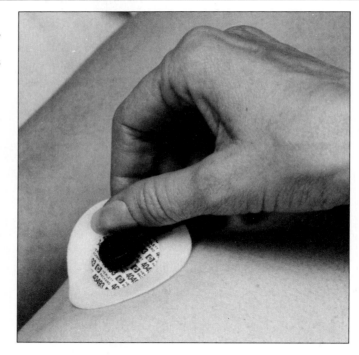

Detecting late potentials

Because late electrical potentials have a low amplitude, you'll need to look closely at a patient's signal-averaged electrocardiogram (ECG) to detect them. Occurring at the end of or just after the QRS complex and lasting from 20 to 60 milliseconds (msec) into the ST segment, late potentials range in amplitude from 1 to 20 microvolts (μV).

Compare the signal-averaged ECGs shown here.

In both examples, the upper tracings reflect cardiac activity from leads Z, X, and Y at high gain; the lower tracings illustrate the filtered QRS complex.

The tracing at left illustrates the absence of late potentials; the tracing at right shows late potentials (see arrow) lasting about 60 msec with a maximum amplitude under 10 μV. The right lower tracing also indicates that the patient has ventricular tachycardia.

Signal-averaged ECG without late potentials

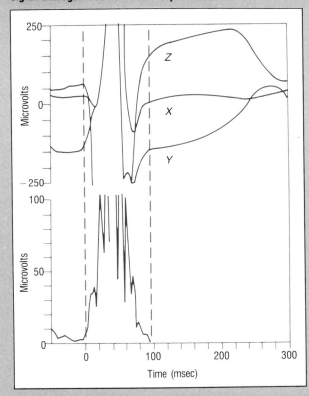

Signal-averaged ECG with late potentials

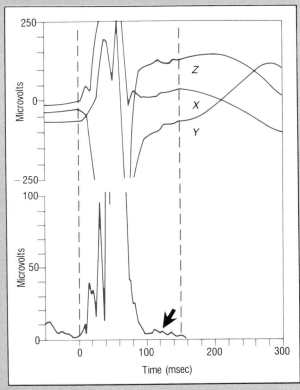

Waveforms provided by Arrhythmia Research Technology, Inc., Austin, Tex.

PATIENT TEACHING

Learning about a signal-averaged electrocardiogram

Dear Patient:

Your doctor has ordered a test called a *signal-averaged electrocardiogram.* This test records the electrical activity of your heart. It uses special computerized equipment to study many of your heartbeats and to create an image of one typical heartbeat. The doctor will then review this typical heartbeat to detect very small electrical signals called *late potentials.* This test can help detect certain heart problems early, when they can be treated most effectively. Here are important steps you can take to make sure that test results are accurate.

What happens before the test
Listen to the nurse's directions about remaining perfectly still when she tells you to. The test takes only a few minutes.

What happens during the test
First, the nurse will clean and rub areas on your chest and back briskly with an alcohol pad. This may redden your skin. If necessary, she may shave the area.

Next, she'll place several small disks called *electrodes* on your skin. She'll attach several electrodes to your chest and one to your back. Then she'll attach thin wires to the electrodes. Don't be concerned: The electrodes will not produce an electric shock.

During the test, keep these directions in mind:
• Remember to lie as still as possible during the test.
• Rest your arms at your sides.
• Don't talk.
• Try to breathe normally.
• Stay relaxed.
• Close your eyes if you want to.
• If you think you have to move, cough, sneeze, or scratch your nose, signal the nurse so that she can stop the test before losing the information that has already been collected. When you feel settled, she'll resume the test.

What happens after the test
Because this test is simple and painless, you won't need any special follow-up care. However, you may feel a minor tugging sensation on your skin when the nurse removes the electrodes.

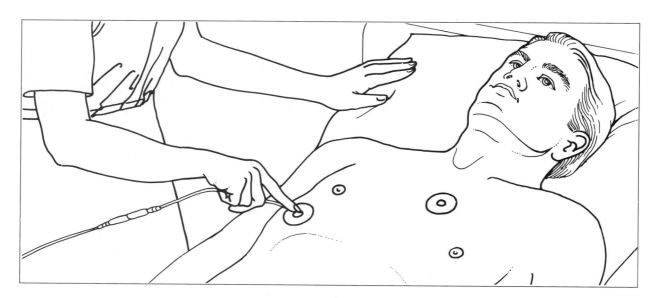

PERFORMING ST-SEGMENT MONITORING

During a 12-lead electrocardiogram (ECG), you may detect ST-segment deviations that require special analysis. To perform this analysis, conduct continuous cardiac monitoring using a 5-lead system; such a system usually allows the best identification of the ST segment. Some bedside cardiac monitors allow ST-segment analysis during continuous monitoring.

A sensitive indicator of myocardial damage, the ST segment is normally flat or isoelectric. A depressed ST segment may result from digitalis glycosides, myocardial ischemia, or a subendocardial infarction. An elevated ST segment suggests myocardial infarction (MI).

Continuous ST-segment monitoring is especially useful for patients who have undergone thrombolytic therapy or coronary angioplasty. Although these procedures help reestablish blood flow to occluded coronary arteries, reocclusion may occur. Monitoring appropriate leads for changes in the ST segment allows early detection of reocclusion.

ST-segment monitoring is also useful for patients who've had previous episodes of cardiac ischemia without chest pain, those who have difficulty distinguishing between cardiac pain and pain from another source (such as arthritis), and those who can't communicate easily.

SELECTING THE BEST LEAD

Because ischemia typically occurs in only one portion of the heart muscle, not all ECG leads detect it; thus, you'll need to select the appropriate leads. One way is to examine ECG tracings recorded during an ischemic episode. For example, if the patient suffered an acute MI, examine both the precordial and limb leads of an ECG recorded before thrombolytic therapy. The leads showing signs of myocardial ischemia during the infarction are the same leads you'll monitor for signs of ischemia in the future.

Also, if the patient has undergone coronary angioplasty, the ECG recorded during the procedure will show you which leads to monitor. Because the balloon catheter inflated during the procedure momentarily obstructs blood flow in the affected coronary artery, ischemia results. The ECG leads that show signs of ischemia are the leads you should monitor for ST-segment changes.

When monitoring the ST segment, keep in mind that the main goal of cardiac monitoring is to detect arrhythmias. Therefore, when deciding which leads to monitor, remember that the leads most likely to reveal arrhythmias should take priority over the leads that may reveal ST-segment changes.

Preparing the equipment and the patient

Begin ST-segment monitoring by collecting the equipment you'll need: ECG electrodes, gauze pads, an ECG monitor cable, leadwires, alcohol sponges (near right), and a cardiac monitor programmed for ST-segment monitoring (such as the Hewlett-Packard Component Monitoring System shown at far right). You may also need a razor.

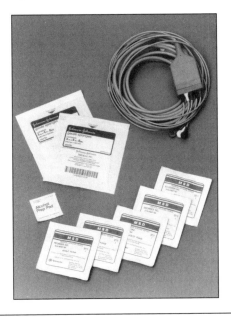
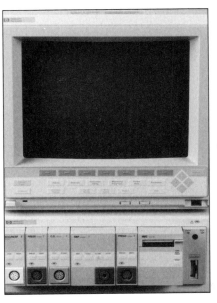

Pamela Kovach, RN, BSN, a clinical consultant for Springhouse Corporation, wrote this section. The publisher thanks *Hewlett-Packard Co.*, Waltham, Mass., and *Hill-Rom*, Batesville, Ind., for their help.

Take the equipment to the patient's bedside and explain the procedure. Then wash your hands. If your patient is not already on a monitor, turn on the device and attach the cable.

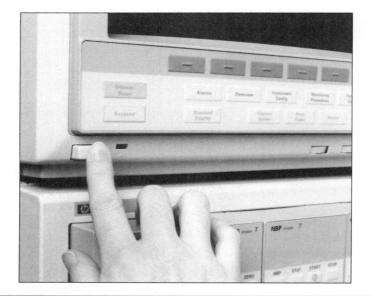

Select the sites for electrode placement according to the lead you'll be monitoring. If necessary, shave the sites. Then clean the sites with an alcohol sponge.

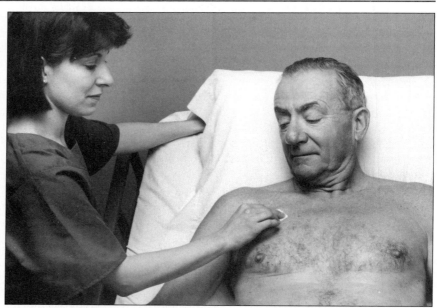

Rub the areas with a gauze pad until the patient's skin becomes red and shiny.

▶ *Clinical tip:* If the electrode has a pumice pad on the back, use it to gently abrade the patient's skin and remove dead skin cells, which will promote electrical conductivity.

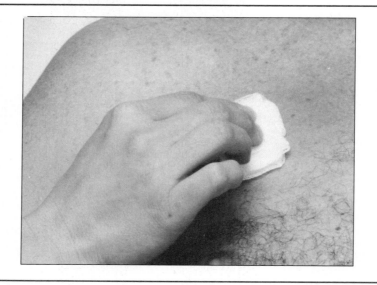

Attach the leadwires to the electrodes.

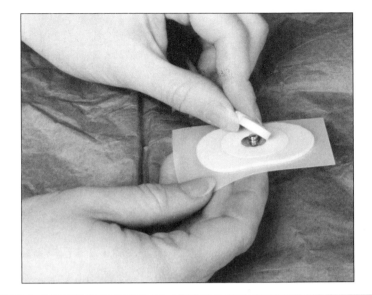

Place the electrodes on the patient's chest in the appropriate positions. For example, the leads at right are placed to record a modified chest lead (MCL$_1$).

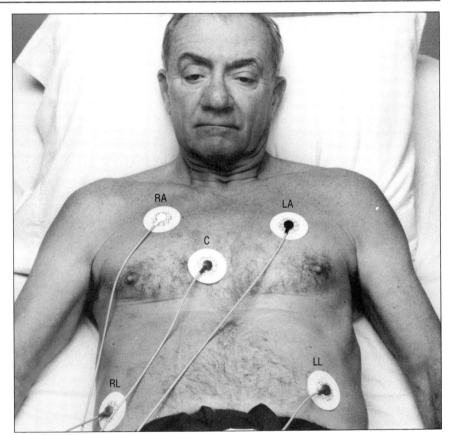

Adjusting the monitor

If necessary, activate ST-segment monitoring by pressing the MONITORING PROCEDURES key and then the ST key (as designated on the screen above the keys).

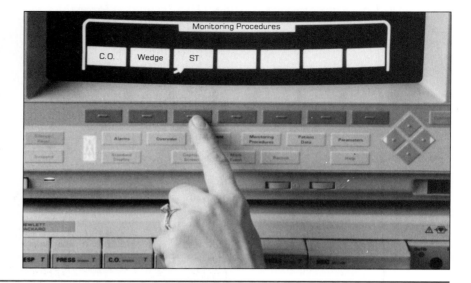

Activate individual ST parameters by pressing the ON/OFF PARAMETER key.

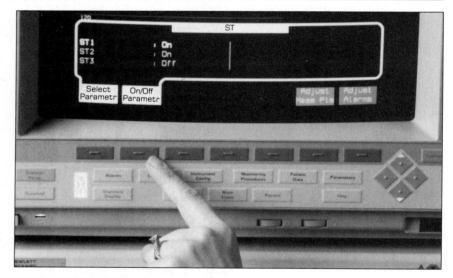

Select the appropriate ECG lead for each ST channel to be monitored by pressing the PARAMETERS key and then the key labeled ECG (as shown).

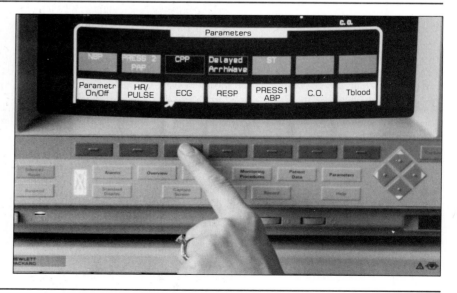

Next, press the key labeled CHANGE LEAD to select the appropriate lead. Repeat the procedure for all three channels.

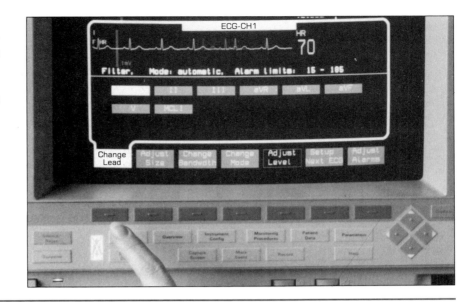 **Clinical tip:** If you monitor only one lead, choose the lead most likely to disclose both arrhythmias and ST-segment changes. Always give precedence, however, to the lead that best shows arrhythmias.

Adjust the ST-segment measurement points, if necessary. To do so, enter the ST task window by pressing the MONITORING PROCEDURES key and then ST. Then press the key labeled ADJUST MEAS PTS.

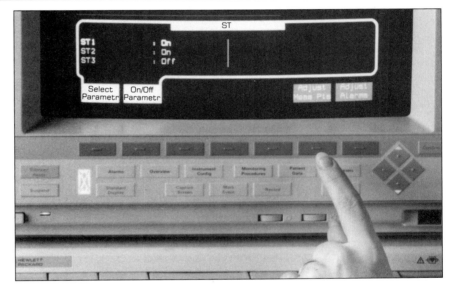

Adjust the baseline for ST-segment measurement, known as the iso-electric point. To do so, press the key marked ISO POINT to move the cursor to the PQ or TP interval (as shown).

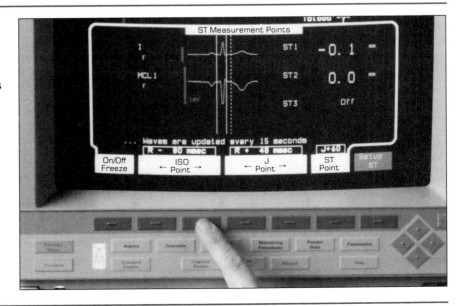

Next, adjust the J point—the transition between the QRS complex and the ST segment. To do so, press the key labeled J POINT to move the cursor to the appropriate location.

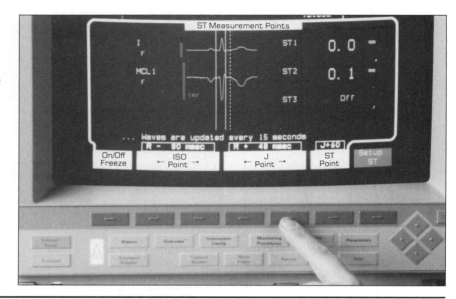

Adjust the ST point to 80 milliseconds after the J point. Do this by pressing the key labeled ST POINT and moving the cursor until the box above the key displays J + 80.

▶ *Clinical tip:* Some hospitals measure the ST point at 60 milliseconds after the J point. Check your hospital's policy before setting the ST point.

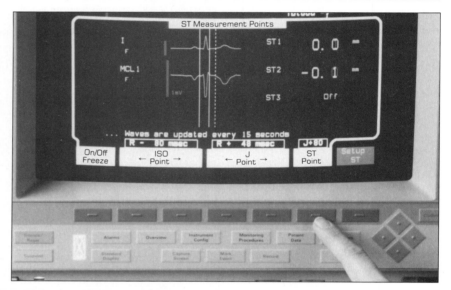

Now set the alarm limits for each ST-segment parameter. First, press the key labeled SETUP ST. Next, press the ADJUST ALARMS key. Then set the high and low limits by manipulating the high and low limit keys (as shown).

▶ *Clinical tip:* The alarms are set according to millimeters of ST-segment depression. When a limit is surpassed for more than 1 minute, both a visual and an audible alarm are activated. Check your hospital's policy, and ask the patient's doctor for alarm limit parameters.

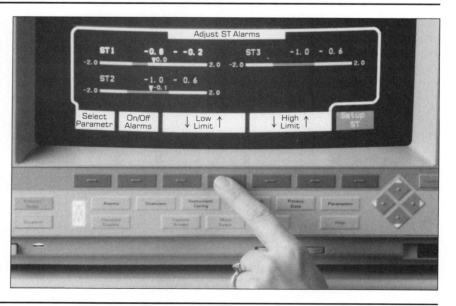

To return to the display screen, press the key labeled STANDARD DISPLAY. If the patient isn't being monitored continuously, remove the electrodes, clean his skin, and disconnect the leadwires from the electrodes.

Document the leads being monitored and the ST-segment measurement points in the patient's chart.

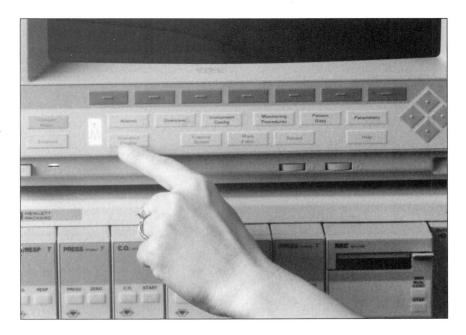

INSIGHTS AND INTERPRETATIONS

Understanding ST-segment elevation and depression

Closely monitoring the ST segment on a patient's electrocardiogram can help you detect ischemia or injury before an infarction develops.

Normal ST segment
The ST segment represents the beginning of ventricular repolarization. It immediately follows the QRS complex (the J point) and extends to the beginning of the T wave. Normally, the ST segment is isoelectric.

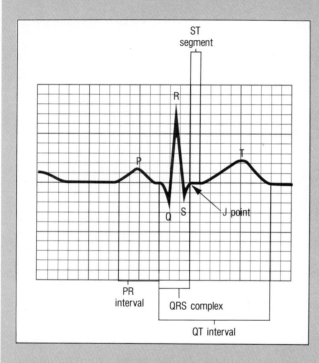

ST-segment depression
A depressed ST segment may indicate myocardial ischemia, subendocardial infarction, or digitalis toxicity. An ST segment is considered depressed when it is 0.5 mm or more from the baseline.

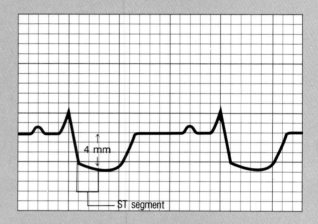

ST-segment elevation
An elevated ST segment may indicate myocardial injury. An ST segment is considered elevated when it is 1 mm or more above the baseline.

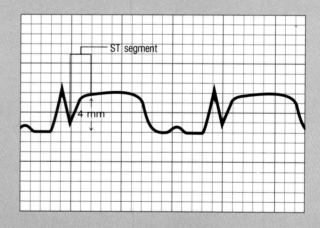

Monitoring Hemodynamic Status

LEARNING ABOUT HEMODYNAMIC MONITORING

Every time you take a patient's blood pressure with a sphygmomanometer, you're performing hemodynamic monitoring. Typically, though, most nurses associate hemodynamic monitoring with invasive procedures used to obtain physiologic measurements from the circulatory system. These procedures permit you to measure cardiac output, central venous pressure (CVP), and intra-arterial pressures, such as pulmonary artery pressure (PAP).

Routinely used in critical care units, invasive hemodynamic monitoring provides accurate, continuous blood pressure readings, even when your patient is in shock. To make the most of hemodynamic monitoring, you need to understand the cardiac cycle, which consists of diastole, when the heart's ventricles fill with blood, and systole, when they contract and eject the blood.

Cardiac cycle

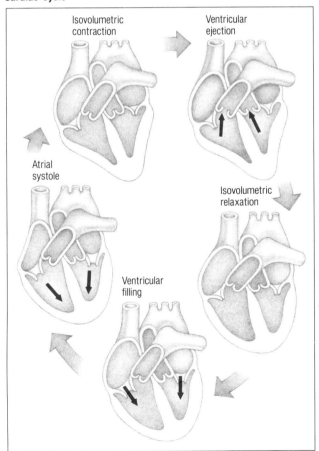

Isovolumetric contraction

Ventricular ejection

Atrial systole

Isovolumetric relaxation

Ventricular filling

This continuous cycle has no set starting point. But for the sake of clarity, assume it begins with isovolumetric contraction and proceeds sequentially through ventricular ejection, isovolumetric relaxation, ventricular filling, and atrial systole.

As depolarization spreads through the ventricles, these chambers contract. The resulting rise in pressure causes the mitral and tricuspid valves to close. Thus, all four heart valves are closed for a short time. The pulmonary and aortic valves stay closed during this phase called *isovolumetric contraction.*

In *ventricular ejection,* ventricular pressure exceeds the aortic and pulmonary arterial pressures. This forces the aortic and pulmonary valves open and permits ejection of ventricular blood.

When ventricular pressure drops below that of the aorta and pulmonary artery, the next phase— *isovolumetric relaxation*—occurs. In this phase, all four heart valves are again closed. At this time, atrial diastole occurs as blood fills the atria.

When the atrial pressure exceeds the ventricular pressure, the mitral and tricuspid valves open. This marks the *ventricular filling* phase in which blood passively enters the ventricles. About 80% of ventricular filling occurs at this time.

The last phase, *atrial systole,* coincides with late diastole, when the atria contract in response to atrial depolarization. This "atrial kick" supplies the ventricles with the remaining 20% of blood before the cycle repeats.

PRESSURE TRANSDUCER SYSTEMS

To perform invasive hemodynamic monitoring, you'll need to be familiar with a pressure transducer system. To operate this device safely and effectively, follow hospital policy and the manufacturer's directions. Keep in mind that sophisticated monitoring techniques can give a false sense of security. Monitoring is just one aspect of nursing care—an adjunct for your clinical judgment.

You'll begin invasive hemodynamic monitoring by setting up a pressure transducer system. This system converts mechanical energy (from blood pressure, for example) into electrical energy (displayed as impulses, or waveforms, on a monitor screen). You'll need this system to monitor arterial pressure, PAP, left atrial pressure, and CVP.

Jan M. Headley, RN, BS, who contributed to this section, is senior education consultant with Baxter Healthcare Corp., Edwards Critical Care Division, Irvine, Calif. The publisher thanks the following organizations for their help: *Baxter Healthcare Corp.,* Irvine, Calif.; *Doylestown (Pa.) Hospital; Hill Rom,* Batesville, Ind.; and *Marquette Electronics,* Milwaukee, Wis.

SETTING UP TRANSDUCERS

The exact type of transducer system you'll set up depends on the patient's needs and the doctor's preference. Some systems monitor pressure continuously, whereas others monitor pressure intermittently. Single-pressure transducers monitor only one type of pressure—for example, PAP. Multiple-pressure transducers can monitor two or more types of pressure, such as PAP and CVP.

Setting up a single-pressure transducer system

Gather the equipment you'll need: monitor; disposable pressure transducer; cable (to connect the pressure transducer to the monitor); preassembled pressure tubing with continuous flush device; inflatable pressure infuser bag; manifold transducer holder (if transducer will be mounted on the I.V. pole); two sterile occlusive (nonvented) caps; a carpenter's level; and a 500-ml bag of heparinized saline solution, commonly called the flush solution bag. Also obtain an I.V. pole.

▶ *Clinical tip:* Adding heparin to a flush solution is controversial. Current studies are investigating whether the system needs heparin to keep the line patent. Keeping this in mind, follow your hospital's policy. If your patient has a history of bleeding or clotting problems, use heparin with caution.

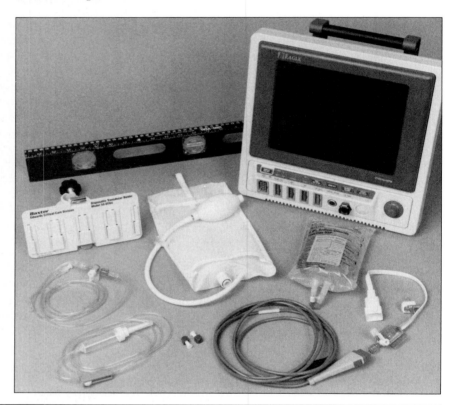

Check the label on the 500-ml bag of heparinized saline solution. Make sure that the patient's name and room number, the date and time, and the amount of added heparin are clearly and correctly labeled. If necessary, add the ordered amount of heparin to the solution—usually, 1 to 2 units of heparin/ml of solution (as shown). Then, label the bag with the appropriate information. (In many hospitals, the pharmacist prepares the flush solution.) Hang the bag that contains the continuous flush solution on the I.V. pole.

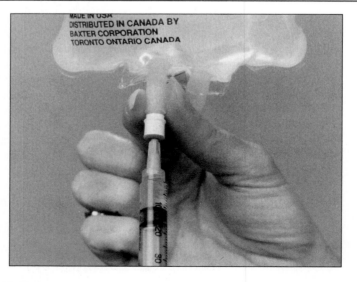

Put the pressure module into the monitor, if necessary, and connect the transducer cable to the monitor. The Marquette Eagle monitor shown here only requires the nurse to attach the transducer cable to the monitor.

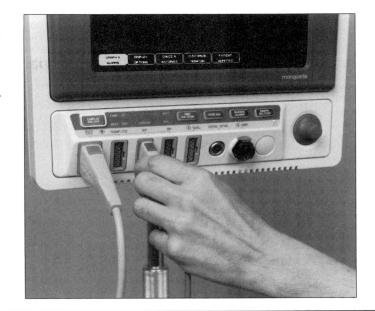

Remove the preassembled pressure tubing from the package. If necessary, connect the pressure tubing to the transducer. Tighten all tubing connections.

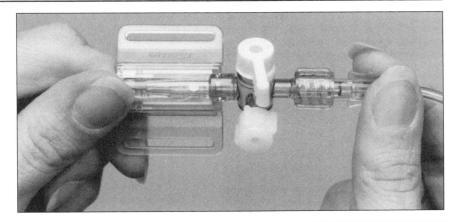

Position all stopcocks so that the flush solution flows through the entire system (near right). Then roll the tubing's flow regulator to the off position (far right).

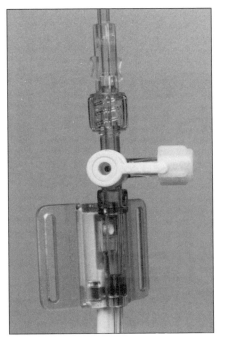
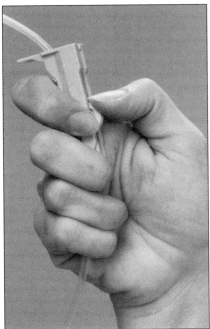

Spike the flush solution bag with the tubing, invert the bag, open the roller clamp, and squeeze all the air through the drip chamber (near right). Then, compress the tubing's drip chamber (far right), filling it no more than halfway with the flush solution.

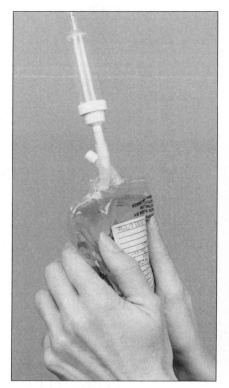
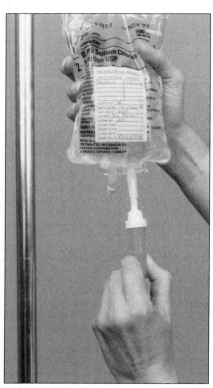

Place the flush solution bag into the pressure infuser bag. To do this, hang the pressure infuser bag on the I.V. pole and then position the flush solution bag inside the pressure infuser bag.

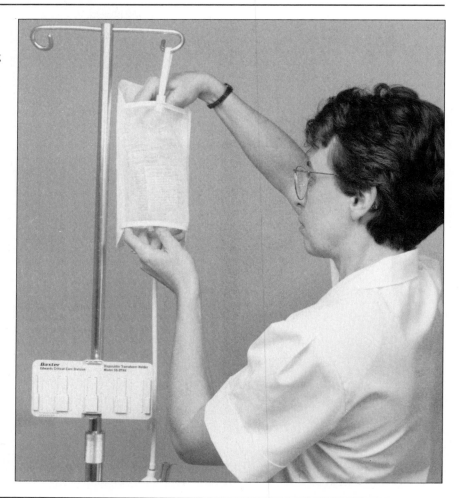

Open the tubing's flow regulator, uncoil the tube if you haven't already done so, and remove the protective cap at the end of the pressure tubing. Squeeze the continuous flush device slowly (as shown) to prime the entire system, including the stopcock ports, with the flush solution.

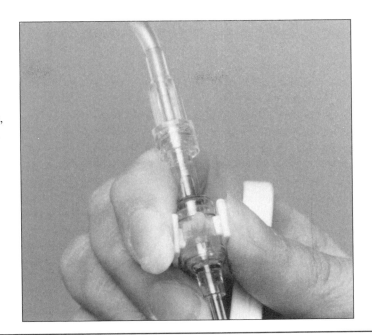

As the solution nears the disposable transducer, hold the transducer at a 45-degree angle. This forces the solution to flow upward to the transducer. In doing so, the solution forces any air out of the system.

▶ *Clinical tip:* As you prime the system, take care to remove all air bubbles—the most common cause of inaccurate pressure readings. Air bubbles may also place the patient at risk for air emboli.

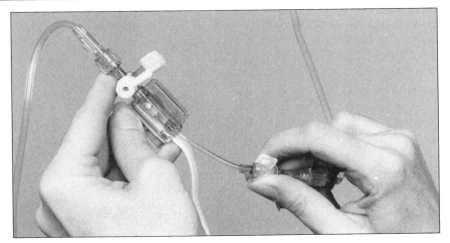

When the solution nears a stopcock, open the stopcock to air, allowing the solution to flow into the stopcock (as shown). When the stopcock fills, close it to air and turn it open to the remainder of the tubing. Do this for each stopcock.

Note: When activated, the continuous flush device allows solution to flow rapidly through the system. When you turn off the continuous flush, the solution's flow rate should be 3 to 5 ml/hour.

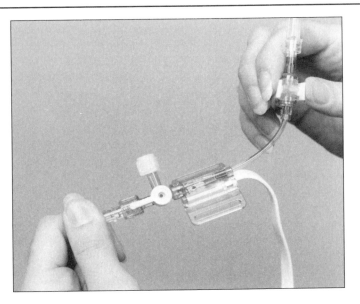

After you completely prime the system, replace the protective cap at the end of the tubing.

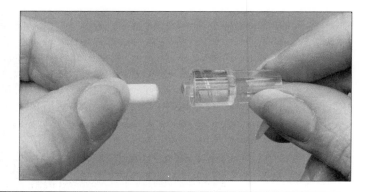

Next, inflate the pressure infuser bag to 300 mm Hg. This bag keeps the pressure in the arterial line higher than the patient's systolic pressure, thereby preventing blood backflow into the tubing and ensuring a continuous flow rate. When you inflate the pressure bag, take care that the drip chamber doesn't completely fill with fluid. Afterward, flush the system again to remove all air bubbles.

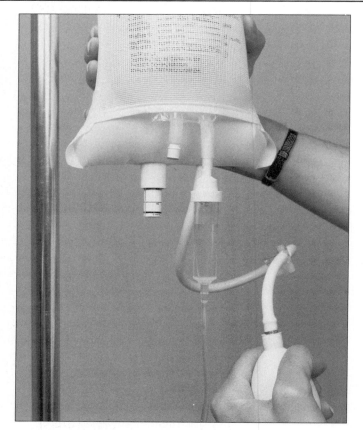

Replace the vented caps on the stopcocks with sterile nonvented caps (near right).

If you're going to mount the transducer on an I.V. pole, insert the device into its holder (far right).

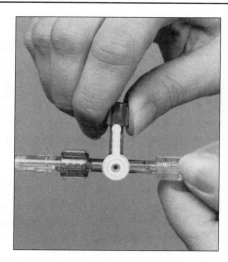

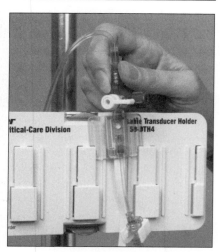

Now you're ready for a preliminary zeroing of the transducer. Zeroing adjusts the transducer so that it reads zero pressure when it's open to the atmosphere. This is important because physiologic pressures, such as arterial blood pressure, are relative to the atmospheric pressure. By zeroing the transducer, you ensure that the device accurately reads pressure within the blood vessel.

▶ **Clinical tip:** To ensure accuracy, position the patient and the transducer on the same level each time you zero the transducer or record a pressure (as shown). Typically, the patient lies flat in bed, if he can tolerate that position.

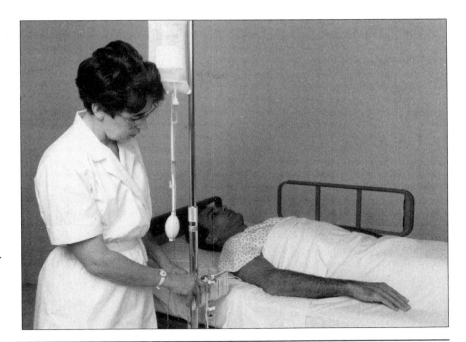

Next, use the carpenter's level to position the air-reference stopcock or the air-fluid interface of the transducer level with the phlebostatic axis (as shown at right). This is also the level of the patient's atria (midway between the posterior chest and his sternum at the fourth intercostal space, midaxillary line, as shown below).

Alternatively, you may level the air-reference stopcock or the air-fluid interface of the transducer to the same position as the catheter tip.

▶ **Clinical tip:** Experts debate the most accurate placement for the transducer. For now, use whichever placement your hospital proposes, and don't vary it.

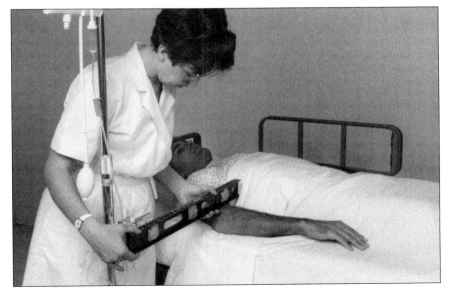

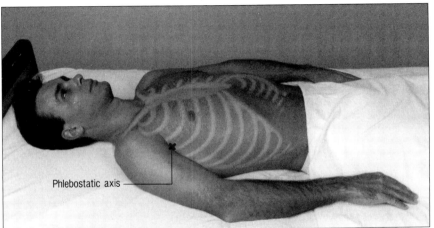

Phlebostatic axis

After leveling the transducer, turn the stopcock next to the transducer *off* to the patient and *open* to air. Remove the cap to the stopcock port. Place the cap inside an opened sterile gauze package to prevent contamination.

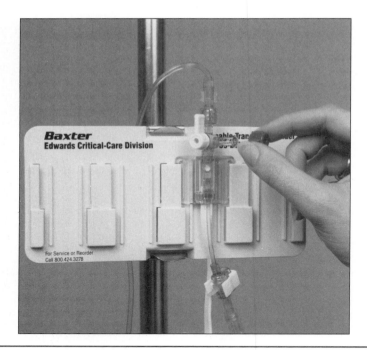

Now, zero the transducer. To do so, follow the manufacturer's direction for zeroing. If you're using the Marquette Eagle monitor shown here, press the ZERO ALL button, and immediately release it. This completes zeroing.

When you've finished zeroing, turn the stopcock on the transducer so that it's *open* to air and *open* to the patient. This is the monitoring position. Replace the cap on the stopcock. You're then ready to attach the single-pressure transducer to the patient's catheter. Document the patient's position for zeroing so that other health care team members can replicate the placement.

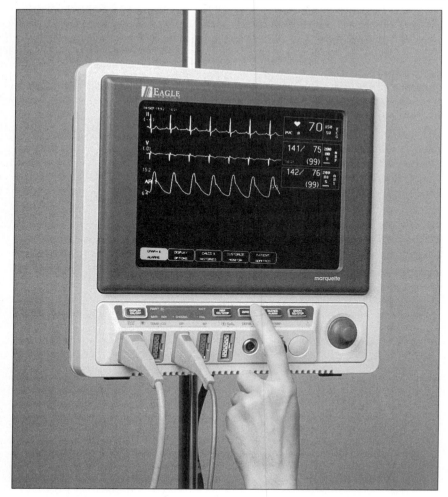

Now, you've assembled a single-pressure transducer system. The photograph at right shows how the system will look.

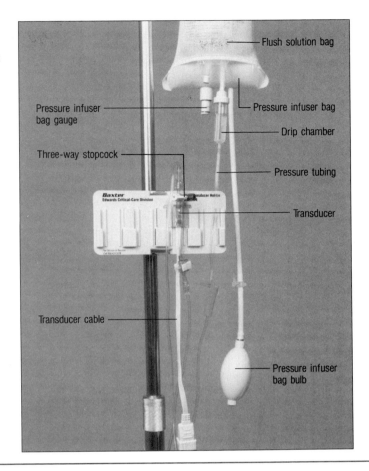

Pressure infuser bag gauge

Three-way stopcock

Transducer cable

Flush solution bag

Pressure infuser bag

Drip chamber

Pressure tubing

Transducer

Pressure infuser bag bulb

Setting up a multiple-pressure transducer system

You may use any of several methods to set up a multiple-pressure transducer system. The equipment you'll need depends on the method you select. But generally, you'll set up another single-pressure transducer system. The two setups make up the multiple-pressure transducer system.

Another way to set up a multiple-pressure transducer system is to assemble equipment as you would for a single-pressure transducer system. But you'll need another cable, and you'll substitute Y-type preassembled pressure tubing with continuous flush devices and two attached pressure transducers for the single-pressure tubing (as shown). You'll also need one more pressure-specific module (if the module isn't built into the cable).

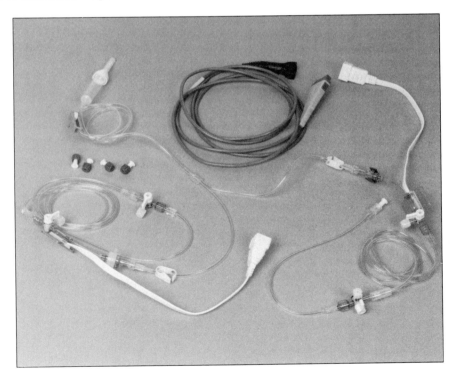

The easiest way to set up a multiple-pressure transducer is to add to the single-pressure system. You'll need another bag of heparinized saline solution in a second pressure infuser bag. Then prime the tubing, mount the second transducer, and connect an additional cable to the monitor. Finally, zero the second transducer, just as you did for the first one.

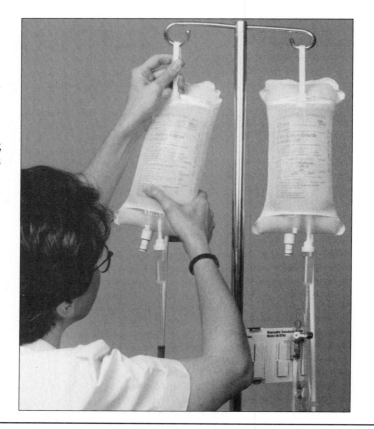

Alternatively, your hospital may use a Y-type tubing setup with two attached pressure transducers. This method requires only one bag of heparinized flush solution. To set up the system, proceed as you would for a single transducer, with this exception: First, prime one branch of the Y-type tubing and then the other. Next, attach two cables to the monitor in the modules for each pressure that you will be measuring. Finally, zero each transducer.

If you need a second pressure reading only intermittently—for example, in continuous PAP monitoring and intermittent CVP monitoring—you may vary the setup by using a transducer with a bridge.

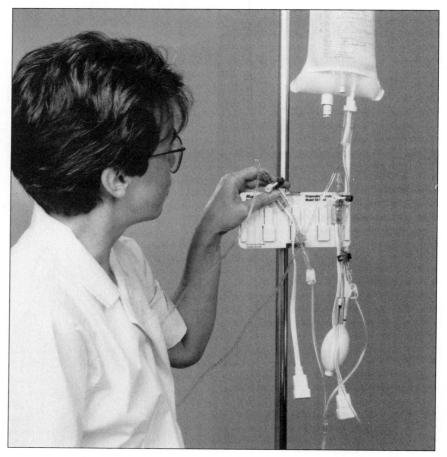

LEARNING ABOUT ARTERIAL PRESSURE MONITORING

Intra-arterial pressure monitoring is used on patients who are severely hypotensive, in shock, or receiving vasoactive medications. And because mean arterial pressure (MAP) helps determine cerebral perfusion pressure, arterial pressure monitoring may also be used when patients have increased intracranial pressure.

HOW ARTERIAL PRESSURE MONITORING WORKS

Typically, the pressure of the patient's arterial pulse wave causes fluid movement in the arterial line tubing, which is connected to a pressure transducer system. The diaphragm of the pressure transducer detects the fluid's motion and converts this mechanical energy into electrical energy.

The resultant signals create a waveform display and a digital printout of the patient's arterial pressure. (See *Understanding the arterial waveform,* below, and *Recognizing abnormal waveforms,* page 86.)

When caring for a patient who has an arterial line, monitor and record:
• systolic pressure (normal range: 100 to 140 mm Hg)
• diastolic pressure (normal range: 60 to 90 mm Hg)
• MAP (normal range: 70 to 105 mm Hg).

In general, *arterial systolic pressure* reflects the peak pressure generated by the left ventricle. It also indicates the compliance of the large arteries—the peripheral resistance.

Arterial diastolic pressure reflects the runoff velocity and the elasticity of the arterial system, particularly the arterioles.

MAP is the average pressure in the arterial system during systole and diastole. It reflects the driving, or perfusion, pressure and is determined by arterial blood volume and blood vessel elasticity and resistance.

To compute MAP, use one of these formulas:
$$MAP = \text{systolic pressure} + 2 (\text{diastolic pressure}) / 3$$
or

$$MAP = \frac{1}{3} \text{ pulse pressure} + \text{diastolic pressure.}$$

Understanding the arterial waveform

Normal arterial blood pressure produces a characteristic waveform, representing ventricular systole and diastole. The waveform has five distinct components: the anacrotic limb, systolic peak, dicrotic limb, dicrotic notch, and end diastole.

The *anacrotic limb* marks the waveform's initial upstroke, which results as blood is rapidly ejected from the ventricle through the open aortic valve into the aorta. The rapid ejection causes a sharp rise in arterial pressure, which appears as the waveform's highest point. This is called the *systolic peak.*

As blood continues into the peripheral vessels, arterial pressure falls, and the waveform begins a downward trend. This part is called *the dicrotic limb.* Arterial pressure usually will continue to fall until pressure in the ventricle is less than pressure in the

aortic root. When this occurs, the aortic valve closes. The event appears as a small notch (the *dicrotic notch*) on the waveform's downside.

When the aortic valve closes, diastole begins, progressing until the aortic root pressure gradually descends to its lowest point. On the waveform, this is known as *end diastole.*

Normal arterial waveform

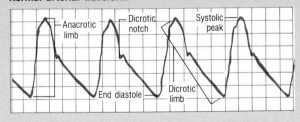

Jan M. Headley, RN, BS, a senior education consultant with Baxter Healthcare Corp., Edwards Critical Care Division, Irvine, Calif., and *Denise Salvo, RN,C, MSN,* clinical faculty member, Widener University, Chester, Pa., contributed to this section. The publisher also thanks the following organizations for their help: *Baxter Healthcare Corp., Edwards Critical Care Division,* Irvine, Calif.; *Doylestown (Pa.) Hospital; Dynatech Nevada,* Carson City, Nev.; *Hewlett Packard,* Waltham, Mass.; and *Hill Rom,* Batesville, Ind.

INSIGHTS AND INTERPRETATIONS

Recognizing abnormal waveforms

Understanding a normal arterial waveform is relatively straightforward. But an abnormal waveform isn't so easy to decipher. Abnormal patterns and markings, however, may provide important diagnostic clues to the patient's cardiovascular status, or they may simply signal trouble in the monitor. Use this chart to help you recognize and resolve waveform abnormalities.

ABNORMALITY	POSSIBLE CAUSES	NURSING INTERVENTIONS
Alternating high and low waves in a regular pattern	• Ventricular bigeminy	• Check the patient's electrocardiogram (ECG) to confirm ventricular bigeminy. The tracing should reflect premature ventricular contractions every second beat.
Flattened waveform	• Overdamped waveform or hypotensive patient	• Check the patient's blood pressure with a sphygmomanometer. If you obtain a reading, suspect overdamping. Correct the problem by trying to aspirate the arterial line. If you succeed, flush the line. If the reading is very low or absent, suspect hypotension.
Slightly rounded waveform with consistent variations in systolic height	• Patient on ventilator with positive end-expiratory pressure	• Check the patient's systolic blood pressure regularly. The difference between the highest and lowest systolic pressure reading should be less than 10 mm Hg. If the difference exceeds that amount, suspect pulsus paradoxus, possibly from cardiac tamponade.
Slow upstroke	• Aortic stenosis	• Check the patient's heart sounds for signs of aortic stenosis. Also notify the doctor, who will document suspected aortic stenosis in his notes.
Diminished amplitude on inspiration	• Pulsus paradoxus, possibly from cardiac tamponade, constrictive pericarditis, or lung disease	• Note systolic pressure during inspiration and expiration. If inspiratory pressure is at least 10 mm Hg less than expiratory pressure, call the doctor. • If you're also monitoring pulmonary artery pressure, observe for a diastolic plateau. This occurs when the mean central venous pressure (right atrial pressure), mean pulmonary artery pressure, and mean pulmonary capillary wedge pressure (pulmonary artery obstructive pressure) are within 5 mm Hg of one another.
Alteration in beat-to-beat amplitude (in otherwise normal rhythm)	• Pulsus alternans, which may indicate left ventricular failure	• Observe the patient's ECG, noting any deviation in the waveform. • Notify the doctor if this is a new and sudden abnormality.

ASSISTING WITH ARTERIAL LINE INSERTION

An arterial line—the access for invasive arterial pressure monitoring—must be inserted by a doctor. Typically, he'll advance a standard 18G to 20G over-the-needle catheter into a peripheral artery, usually the radial, brachial, or femoral artery. The radial artery is preferred. (See *Choosing an arterial catheter site.*) The line is known commonly as an "art" or "A" line.

Before accessing the radial artery, however, you'll check the patient's ulnar and radial circulation. Why? If the radial artery is blocked by a blood clot (a common complication of arterial lines), the ulnar artery alone must supply blood to the hand. A simple, reliable test of circulation can be done by performing Allen's test, which demonstrates how well both arteries supply blood to the hand.

Choosing an arterial catheter site

When your patient needs hemodynamic monitoring, the doctor will probably insert an arterial catheter in a radial or brachial artery. If these sites are unsuitable, he may insert the catheter in the femoral or dorsalis pedis artery. Here are some advantages and disadvantages to consider for each insertion site.

INSERTION SITE	ADVANTAGES	DISADVANTAGES
Radial artery	• This site is easy to locate. • The ulnar artery provides good collateral circulation to the hand. • The site is easy to observe and maintain. • The area is anatomically stable; the radius acts as a natural splint.	• The artery has a relatively small lumen, so catheter insertion may be difficult and painful. • Pressure readings may be false-high because of the site's distance from the heart.
Brachial artery	• This artery is larger than the radial artery and easily located. • The site is easy to observe and maintain. • Bleeding can usually be prevented or controlled by direct pressure. • Pressure readings may be more accurate because of the site's proximity to the heart.	• Median nerve damage is possible during catheter insertion. • Tissue damage may occur if the artery occludes because of inadequate collateral circulation to the lower arm. • To stabilize the catheter, the patient's elbow must be splinted. This may produce joint stiffness. • Thrombosis may occur if the artery is small (in children and small women) or if the patient has low cardiac output.
Femoral artery	• With its large lumen, this vessel may be the easiest artery to locate and puncture during an emergency. • The site is anatomically stable; the femur acts as a natural splint.	• Catheter insertion may damage the nearby femoral vein and major nerves. • The site poses a high risk of thrombosis. • If the artery occludes, tissue damage is possible because of inadequate collateral circulation. • The catheter is difficult to secure at this site. • Bleeding at this site is difficult to prevent or control. • The insertion site is difficult to bandage and keep clean.
Dorsalis pedis artery	• This site may be used when other sites can't be used because of burns or other injuries.	• The site poses a high risk of thrombosis.

As with other invasive hemodynamic monitoring techniques, you'll need to set up a pressure transducer system such as the one shown at right. You'll also need an I.V. pole.

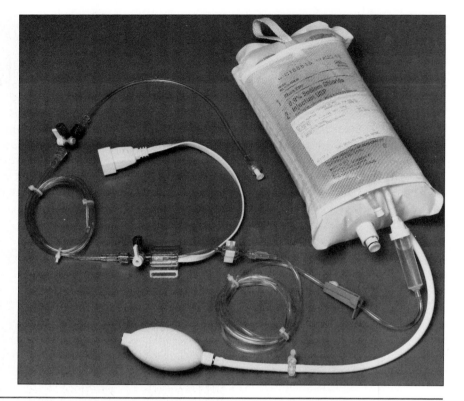

Additional supplies include sterile gloves (two pairs: one for the doctor, one for you); a local anesthetic (such as 1% lidocaine, as ordered by the doctor); a 2″ 18G or 20G over-the-needle catheter; a 3-ml syringe with 23G needle for the local anesthetic; povidone-iodine solution applicator; a linen-saver pad; nonallergenic tape; antimicrobial ointment; dry, sterile dressings for the access site, such as 3″ × 3″ or 4″ × 4″ gauze pads or a transparent dressing, according to hospital policy; a carpenter's level; and an armboard. You'll also need a monitor with arterial pressure capabilities.

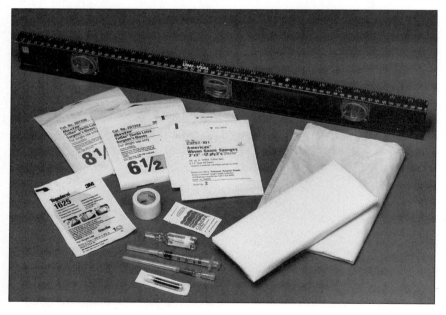

Bring the prepared pressure transducer system to the patient's room, and hang it on an I.V. pole. Insert the arterial pressure module into the monitor if it's not already in place and if you'll be using the manifold mount. Attach the mount to the I.V. pole if it's not already in place, and put the transducer into the mount. Alternatively, you can mount the transducer on the patient's arm. Next, connect the transducer cable to the monitor (as shown). Then level and zero the transducer. (See "Setting up transducers" earlier in this section.)

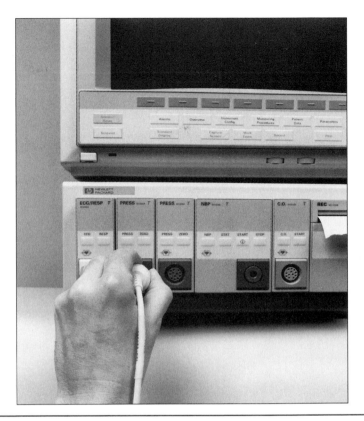

Explain the procedure to the patient. Reassure her that the doctor will use a local anesthetic to minimize discomfort. Position her comfortably, but make sure that the insertion site is level and easily accessible.

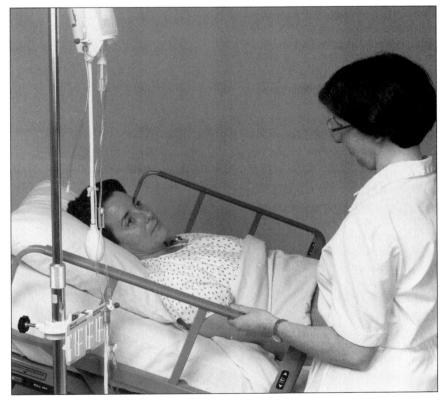

If the radial artery will be used, perform Allen's test now. Elevate the patient's hand, and have her clench and unclench this hand. Next, have her rest her arm. Then, slide a rolled towel under her wrist for support. Ask her to clench her fist while you compress her radial and ulnar arteries for about 1 minute with your fingers. Then, lower her hand.

▶ *Clinical tip:* If your patient can't clench and unclench her hand, assess collateral circulation. Get her palm to blanch by occluding both arteries, elevating her hand, and massaging her palm.

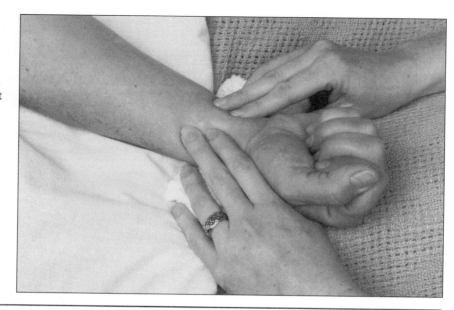

Next, lower the patient's hand. Without removing your fingers from the arteries, ask her to unclench her fist and relax her hand. The palm will appear pale because you've impaired the normal blood flow with your fingers.

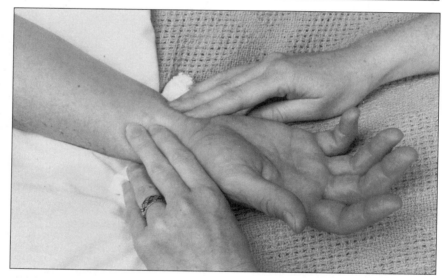

Release the pressure on the ulnar artery, but keep pressure on the radial artery. Observe the palm for a brisk return of color, which should occur within 7 seconds (showing a patent ulnar artery and adequate blood flow to the hands). If color returns in 7 to 15 seconds, blood flow is impaired; if color returns after 15 seconds, consider the flow inadequate.

If blood flow is impaired or inadequate, the radial artery shouldn't be used. At this point, proceed with Allen's test in the other hand. If neither hand colors, the doctor may insert the catheter via the brachial artery.

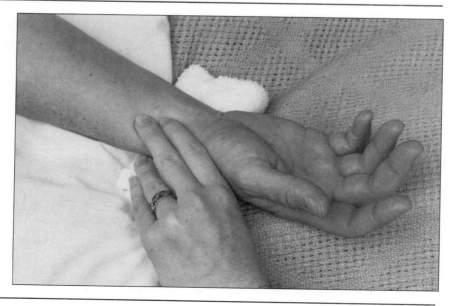

Place a linen-saver pad under the insertion site, and position the site so that it's accessible and easily visible (as shown). Put on sterile gloves and place a sterile towel over the linen-saver pad. The doctor will clean the site, using the povidone-iodine solution applicator (or an equivalent cleaning agent according to hospital policy). As needed, help the doctor prepare the site and perform the procedure.

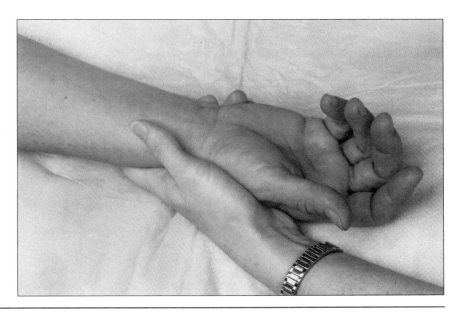

As the insertion nears completion, remove the protective cap from the end of the prepared pressure tubing.

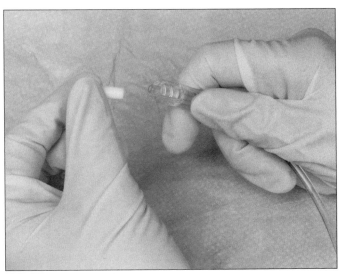

Fast-flush the tubing and, as the doctor stabilizes the catheter hub, immediately connect the tubing to the catheter hub. Fast flushing helps prevent air from entering the system when you connect the tubing to the catheter.

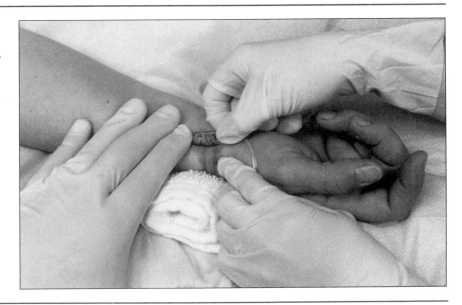

After you connect the tubing, check to make sure that the patient's arterial waveform appears on the monitor.

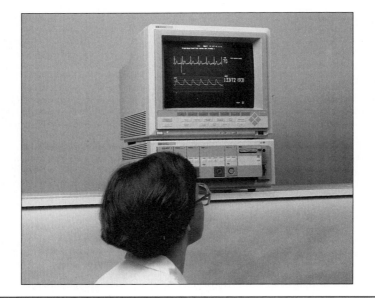

As soon as a proper waveform appears, the doctor will suture the catheter in place. Then either the doctor or nurse (in this instance, the nurse) applies an antibiotic ointment to the site and covers it with a dressing, according to hospital policy. A transparent dressing or 3″ × 3″ or 4″ × 4″ gauze pads and nonallergenic tape (shown here) may be used.

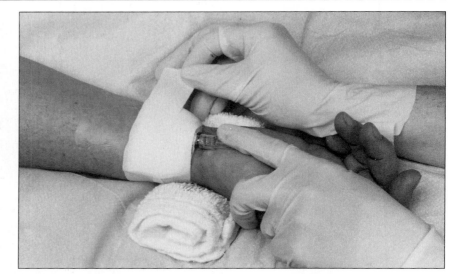

If you applied the dressing, you'll next need to level and zero the transducer. (If the doctor applies the dressing and the transducer is already mounted on the I.V. pole, you can relevel and rezero it while the doctor dresses the catheter site.) You can remove your gloves before this step, if you wish.

Now, recheck the configuration of the arterial waveform. A crisp tracing indicates accurate placement.

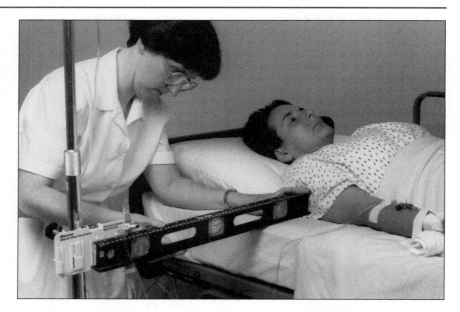

If the transducer is placed on the patient's forearm, loop the pressure tubing around the patient's thumb and attach the transducer, using the strap provided, to her forearm above the catheter insertion site.

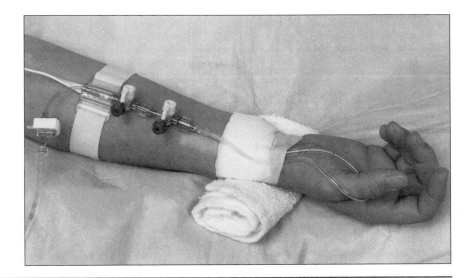

Carefully set the monitor alarms at 20 mm Hg above and below the patient's desired arterial pressure readings. Then measure and record the systolic, diastolic, and mean arterial pressures.

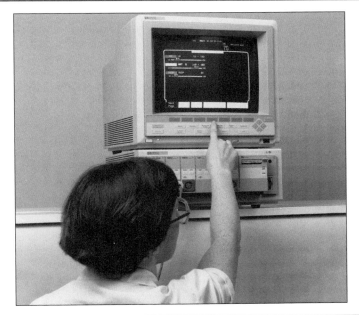

Next, secure the pressure tubing and catheter. To do this, position the patient's hand on an armboard with the palm side up. If needed, place a roll of dressing material or a rolled washcloth under the wrist.

▶ *Clinical tip:* Take care not to hyperextend or dorsiflex the wrist because this can cause neuromuscular injury to the hand or dislodge the catheter.

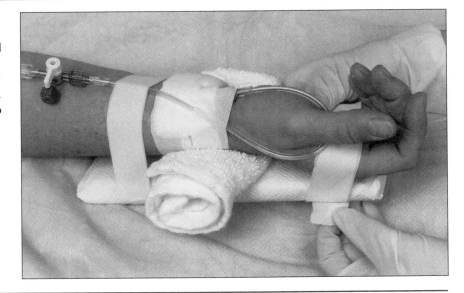

Make sure that the patient's arm is over her bed covers. Instruct her to keep her hand above the covers so that it's easily visible.

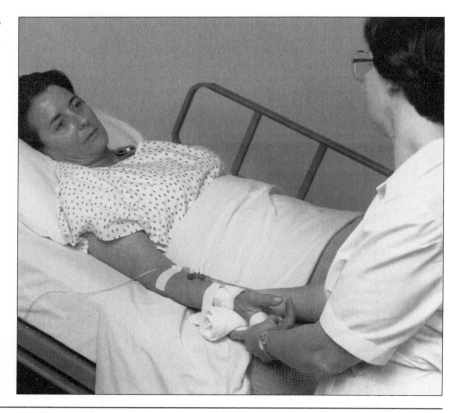

Check the circulation in the patient's hand at least once every 2 hours. Have her tell you if she has any tingling, pain, or numbness in that area. Finally, document the procedure.

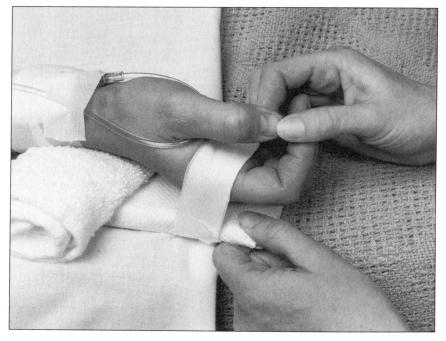

MANAGING AN ARTERIAL LINE

Once the patient's arterial line is secure and the monitor is set up, you'll need to monitor the arterial line and check the system frequently to ensure accurate pressure readings and the patient's comfort and safety. When caring for a patient's arterial line, always use sterile technique, and always observe electrical safety precautions.

Managing an arterial line consists of several patient care procedures, such as taking a cuff pressure, replacing the flush solution, changing both the flush solution and the pressure tubing, and obtaining a blood sample. The type of equipment you'll need depends on which procedure you're performing. (See *Equipment for arterial line management.*)

Equipment for arterial line management

What equipment do you need to manage your patient's arterial line? It all depends on which procedure you're doing. For the procedures noted below, you'll need the pictured items.

Assessing cuff pressure
• Blood pressure cuff and stethoscope

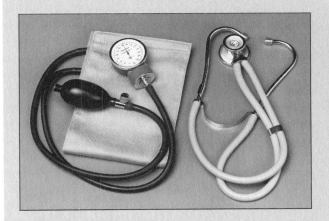

Replacing the flush solution
• A 500-ml bag of heparinized saline solution

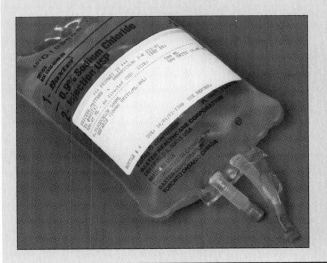

Changing the flush solution and pressure tubing
• Gloves and prepared pressure transducer system

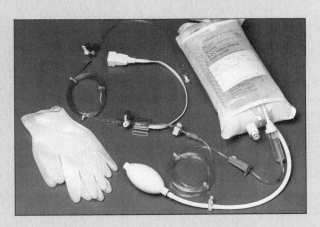

Drawing a blood sample
• Gloves, two 5-ml syringes, 20G needle, various color-top laboratory test tubes, and several 3″ × 3″ or 4″ × 4″ sterile gauze pads

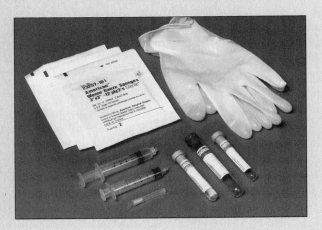

Performing routine assessment and taking a cuff pressure

Monitor the patient's arterial pressure, and assess the appearance of her arterial waveform hourly—or more often if necessary. Also, read and record the digital display of blood pressure values on the monitor, and notify the doctor of any significant changes.

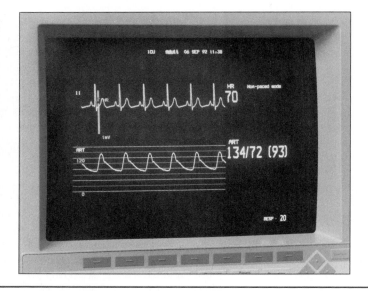

Compare the arterial line pressure with the cuff pressure as often as your hospital policy dictates, but at least once each shift. Expect the direct arterial pressure to be 5 to 15 mm Hg higher than the blood pressure cuff measurement. At the beginning of each shift and after any manipulation of the patient or the system, level and zero the system (see "Setting up transducers" earlier in this section).

▶ *Clinical tip:* Remember, a series of blood pressure measurements over time provides more reliable clinical information than a single isolated measurement.

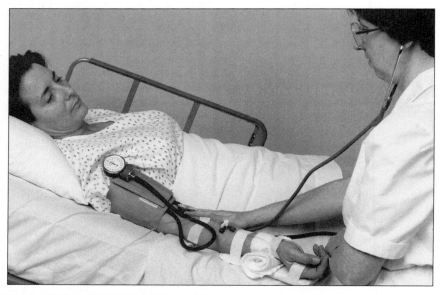

Every 2 to 4 hours, assess the patient's hand on the cannulated side, noting skin color, temperature, and circulation. Also check to ensure that the patient has sensation in the cannulated extremity distal to the insertion site. If the patient states that she's experiencing numbness or tingling (signs of neurovascular compromise), notify the doctor.

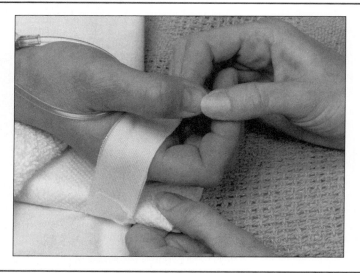

Double-check the integrity of the monitoring system. Be sure to position all stopcocks properly.

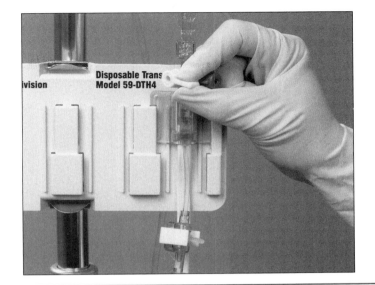

Also be sure to secure all connections (as shown). As you do this, check the waveform for damping and the pressure line to ensure that no air has entered the system.

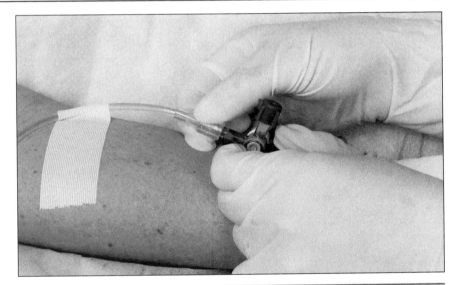

Maintain arterial line patency by flushing the line periodically. Be careful to avoid using excessive pressure, which could cause arteriospasms.

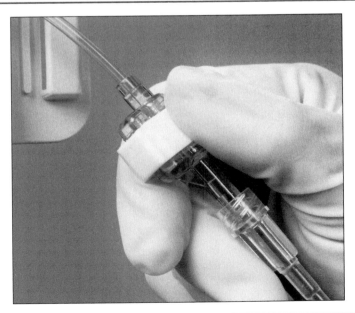

Replacing the flush solution

You may need to replace the flush solution if the flush solution bag leaks or if the I.V. tubing spike is inadvertently disconnected from the flush solution bag. Begin by turning the stopcock off to the patient. This prevents blood from flowing back into the tubing.

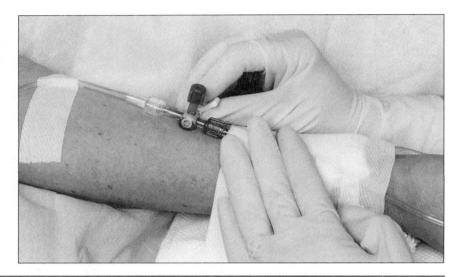

Roll the tubing's flow regulator to the off position.

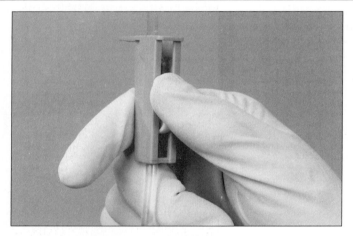

Deflate the pressure infuser bag by opening the valve near the bulb (as shown near right). Then remove the flush solution from the bag (as shown far right).

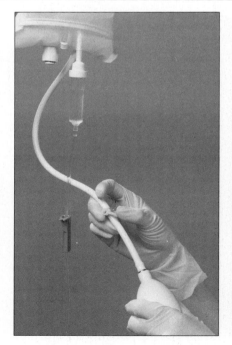
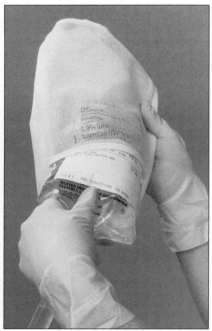

Disconnect the used heparinized flush solution bag, and attach the fresh heparinized flush solution bag to the pressure tubing. Then invert the bag and squeeze it. This forces any air in the bag out through the tubing. Throughout the procedure, take care not to introduce air into the system.

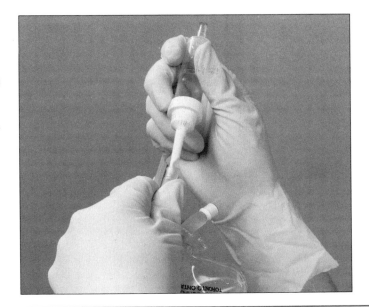

Compress the drip chamber on the new bag until the chamber fills halfway with the flush solution (as shown near right). Then put the bag into the pressure infuser bag, hang the bag on the I.V. pole, and inflate the pressure infuser bag to 300 mm Hg (as shown far right).

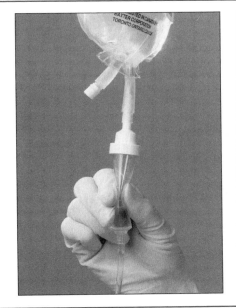
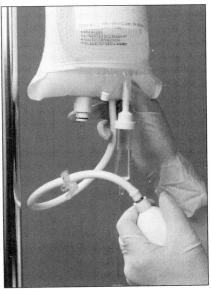

Next, open the pressure tubing's flow regulator and flush the tubing with the new solution. Hold a sterile gauze pad under each stopcock port to catch the expelled solution.

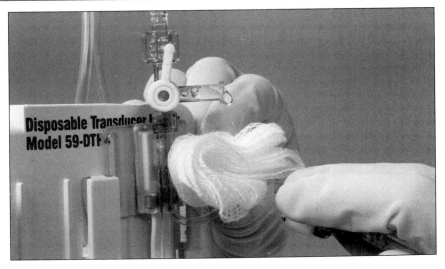

After you've removed all the air, turn each stopcock so that the system is open to the patient (as shown). Replace the occlusive caps on the stopcock ports. If necessary, flush any blood from the tubing.

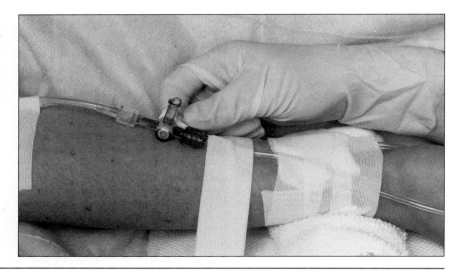

Changing the flush solution and the pressure tubing

As directed by your hospital policy, you'll need to change both the flush solution and the pressure tubing periodically, usually every 48 hours. First, prepare a new pressure transducer system (as described in "Setting up transducers" earlier in this section). Then place a linen-saver pad under the patient's forearm, and put on gloves.

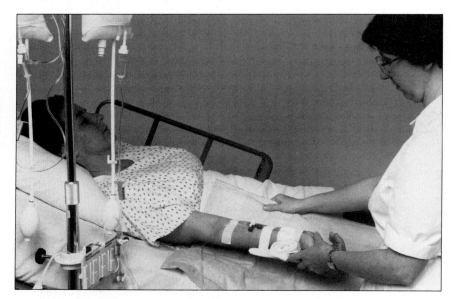

Remove the dressings over the site and examine the site. Next, flush the old system. Then, as you apply pressure to the artery, disconnect the old tubing and quickly screw the new tubing into the catheter hub (as shown). You may want someone to assist by stabilizing the catheter hub as you connect the new tubing. Tighten all connections and redress the site.

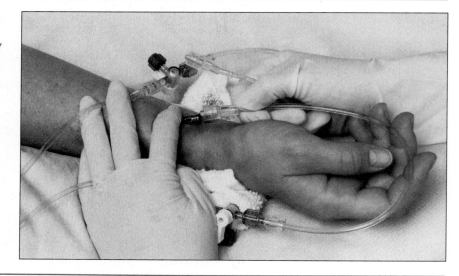

Flush the new system, and attach the transducer cable to the new transducer.

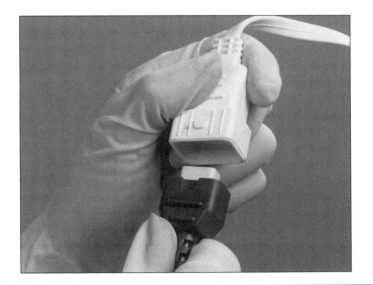

Finally, level and zero the new transducer. Watch for the waveform to appear on the monitor.

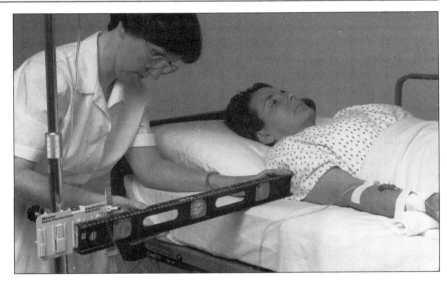

Obtaining a blood sample from an arterial line

Assemble your equipment, wash your hands, and put on gloves. Next, turn off the alarms. Remove the occlusive cap from the stopcock closest to the patient and place it on a 3″ × 3″ or 4″ × 4″ sterile gauze pad. Then insert a 5-ml syringe into the stopcock. Turn the stopcock off to the flush solution and open to the sampling port. Slowly withdraw 3 to 5 ml of blood from the line.

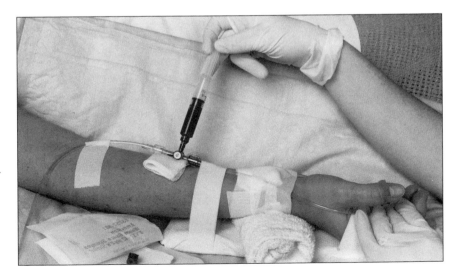

Turn the stopcock halfway back so that it's open to the patient. (This will close the system in all directions.) Finally, remove the syringe and discard this blood according to hospital policy.

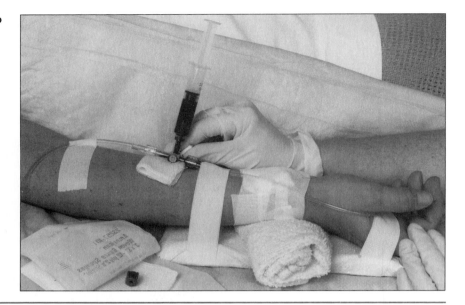

Attach a fresh, sterile 5-ml syringe to the stopcock. Turn the stopcock so that it's open to the sampling port, and draw blood into the syringe. Again, turn the stopcock to the halfway position. Remove the syringe. Attach a 20G needle, and inject the blood into the appropriate color-top tube for the ordered test (as shown).

Then turn the stopcock off to the patient and open to the sampling port. Flush the line. Hold a gauze pad under the port to collect the expelled solution.

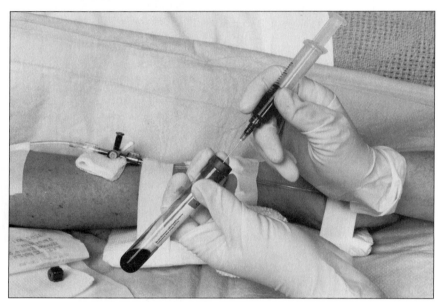

After clearing the port, turn the stopcock off to the port and open to the patient. Reapply the cap to the stopcock port, and flush the entire system. Check to make sure that the waveform is correct, and turn on the alarms. Finally, document the procedure.

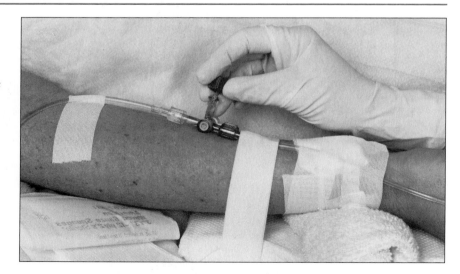

TROUBLESHOOTING

Dealing with problems of arterial lines

When you care for a patient with an arterial line, several problems may interfere with proper functioning of the setup or your ability to interpret a waveform. This chart outlines causes and solutions to some of the most common problems.

PROBLEM	CAUSE	SOLUTION
Damped waveform Appearing as a small waveform with a slow rise in the anacrotic limb and a reduced or nonexistent dicrotic notch, a damped waveform may result from interference with transmission of the physiologic signal to the transducer.	• Air in the system	• Check the system for air, paying particular attention to the tubing and the transducer's diaphragm. If you find air, aspirate it or force it from the system through a stopcock port. Never flush any fluid containing air bubbles into the patient.
	• Loose connection	• Check and tighten all connections.
	• Clotted catheter tip	• Attempt to aspirate the clot. If you're successful, flush the line. If you're not successful, avoid flushing the line; you could dislodge the clot.
	• Catheter tip resting against the arterial wall	• Reposition the catheter insertion area—usually the wrist—and flush the catheter. Or reposition the catheter by carefully rotating it or pulling it back slightly.
	• Kinked tubing	• Unkink the tubing.
	• Inadequately inflated pressure infuser bag	• Inflate the pressure infuser bag to 300 mm Hg.
Drifting waveform Waveform floats above and below the baseline.	• Temperature change in the flush solution	• Allow the temperature of the flush solution to stabilize before infusing it.
	• Kinked or compressed monitor cable	• Check the cable and relieve the kink or compression.
Inability to flush the arterial line or to withdraw blood Activating the continuous flush device fails to move the flush solution, and blood can't be withdrawn from the stopcock.	• Incorrectly positioned stopcocks	• Properly reposition the stopcocks.
	• Kinked tubing	• Unkink the tubing.
	• Inadequately inflated pressure infuser bag	• Inflate the pressure infuser bag to 300 mm Hg.
	• Clotted catheter tip	• Attempt to aspirate the clot. If you're successful, flush the line. If you're not successful, avoid flushing the line; you could dislodge the clot.
	• Catheter tip resting against the arterial wall	• Reposition the catheter insertion area, and flush the catheter. Or reposition the catheter by carefully rotating it or pulling it back slightly.
	• Position of the insertion area	• Check the position of the insertion area, and change it as indicated. For radial and brachial arterial lines, use an armboard to immobilize the area. With a femoral arterial line, keep the head of the bed at a 45-degree angle or less to prevent catheter kinking.
Artifact Waveform tracings follow an erratic pattern or fail to appear as a recognizable diagnostic pattern.	• Electrical interference	• Check electrical equipment in the room.
	• Patient movement	• Ask the patient to lie quietly while you try to read the monitor.
	• Catheter whip or fling (excessive catheter tip movement)	• Shorten the tubing, if possible.

(continued)

Dealing with problems of arterial lines *(continued)*

PROBLEM	CAUSE	SOLUTION
False-high pressure reading Arterial pressure exceeds the patient's normal pressure without a significant change in baseline clinical findings. Before responding to this high pressure, recheck the system to make sure that the reading is accurate.	• Improper calibration	• Recalibrate the system.
	• Transducer positioned below the phlebostatic axis or as indicated	• Relevel the transducer with the phlebostatic axis or as indicated.
	• Catheter kinked	• Unkink the catheter.
	• Clotted catheter tip	• Attempt to aspirate the clot. If you're successful, flush the line. If you're not successful, avoid flushing the line; you could dislodge the clot.
	• Catheter tip resting against the arterial line	• Flush the catheter, or reposition it by carefully rotating it or pulling it back slightly.
	• I.V. tubing too long	• Shorten the tubing by removing extension tubing (if used), or replace the administration set with a set that has shorter tubing.
	• Small air bubbles in tubing close to patient	• Remove air bubbles.
False-low pressure reading Arterial pressure drops below the patient's normal pressure without a significant change in baseline clinical findings. Before responding to this low pressure, recheck the system to ensure that the reading is accurate.	• Improper calibration	• Recalibrate the system.
	• Transducer positioned above the level of the phlebostatic axis or as indicated	• Relevel the transducer with the phlebostatic axis or as indicated.
	• Loose connections	• Check and tighten all connections.
	• Catheter kinked	• Unkink the catheter.
	• Clotted catheter tip	• Attempt to aspirate the clot. If you're successful, flush the line. If you're not successful, avoid flushing the line; you could dislodge the clot.
	• Catheter tip resting against the arterial line	• Reposition the catheter insertion area, and flush the catheter. Or reposition the catheter by carefully rotating it or pulling it back slightly.
	• I.V. tubing too long	• Shorten the tubing by removing the extension tubing (if used), or replace the administration set with a set having shorter tubing.
	• Large air bubble close to the transducer	• Reprime the transducer.
No waveform No waveform appears on the monitor.	• No power supply	• Turn on the power.
	• Loose connections	• Check and tighten all connections.
	• Stopcocks turned off to the patient	• Position the stopcocks properly. Make sure that the transducer is open to the catheter.
	• Transducer disconnected from the monitor module	• Reconnect the transducer to the monitor module.
	• Occluded catheter tip	• Attempt to aspirate the clot. If you're successful, flush the line. If you're not successful, avoid flushing the line; you could dislodge the clot.
	• Catheter tip resting against the arterial wall	• Flush the catheter, or reposition it by carefully rotating it or pulling it back slightly.

COMPLICATIONS

Minimizing risks of arterial lines

For most critically ill patients, the advantages of arterial lines overcome the disadvantages. However, because any invasive hemodynamic monitoring procedure poses some risk, you'll need to watch your patient for complications that may result from an arterial line. This summary of major complications covers causes, effective responses, and tips for prevention.

COMPLICATIONS AND SIGNS AND SYMPTOMS	POSSIBLE CAUSES	NURSING INTERVENTIONS	PREVENTION
Thrombosis • Loss or weakening of pulse below arterial line insertion site • Loss of warmth, sensation, and mobility in limb below insertion site • Damped or straight waveform on monitor display or printout	• Arterial damage during or after insertion • Sluggish flush solution flow rate • Failure to heparinize flush solution adequately • Failure to flush catheter routinely and after withdrawing blood samples • Irrigation of clotted catheter with a syringe	• Notify the doctor. He may remove the line. • Document the complication and record your interventions.	• Check the patient's pulse rate immediately after catheter insertion, then once hourly. • Reduce injury to the artery by splinting the limb holding the line and by taping the catheter securely. • Check the flush solution's flow rate hourly; maintain the rate at 3 to 4 ml/hour. • Heparinize the flush solution according to hospital policy. • Flush the catheter once hourly and after withdrawing blood samples. • Never irrigate an arterial catheter. You may flush a blood clot into the bloodstream.
Blood loss • Bloody dressing; blood flowing from disconnected line	• Dislodged catheter • Disconnected line	• Stop the bleeding. • Check the patient's vital signs. • Notify the doctor if blood loss is great or if the patient's vital signs change. • If the line is disconnected, avoid reconnecting it. Instead, immediately replace contaminated equipment. • If the catheter is pulled out of the vein, remove it and apply direct pressure to the site; then notify the doctor. • When the bleeding stops, check the patient's pulse and the insertion site frequently for signs of thrombosis or hematoma. • Document the complication and your interventions.	• Check the line connections and insertion site frequently. • Tape the catheter securely and splint the patient's limb.
Air embolism or thromboembolism • Drop in blood pressure • Rise in central venous pressure • Weak, rapid pulse • Cyanosis • Loss of consciousness • Damped waveform	• Air in tubing • Loose connections	• Place the patient on his left side and in Trendelenburg's position. If air has entered the heart chambers, this position may keep the air on the heart's right side. The pulmonary artery can then absorb the small air bubbles. • Check the arterial line for leaks. • Notify the doctor immediately, and check the patient's vital signs. • Administer oxygen, if ordered. • Document the complication and your interventions.	• Expel all air from the line before connecting it to the patient. • Make sure that all connections are secure; then check connections routinely. • Change the flush solution bag before it empties. • Prevent thromboembolism by keeping the arterial line patent with heparinized flush solution.

(continued)

Minimizing risks of arterial lines *(continued)*

COMPLICATIONS AND SIGNS AND SYMPTOMS	POSSIBLE CAUSES	NURSING INTERVENTIONS	PREVENTION
Systemic infection • Sudden rise in temperature and pulse rate • Chills and shaking • Blood pressure changes	• Poor aseptic technique • Equipment contaminated during manufacture, storage, or use • Irrigation of clotted catheter	• Look for other sources of infection first. Obtain urine, sputum, and blood specimens for cultures and other analyses, as ordered. • Notify the doctor. He may discontinue the line and send the equipment to the laboratory for study. • Document the complication and record your interventions.	• Review care procedures and ensure aseptic technique. • Take care not to contaminate the arterial line insertion site when bathing the patient. • If any part of the line disconnects accidentally, don't rejoin it. Instead, replace the parts with sterile equipment. • Change system components as recommended: I.V. flush solution and pressure tubing every 48 hours, transparent dressing every 7 days, nontransparent dressing every 24 to 48 hours, and catheter every 72 hours.
Arterial spasm • Intermittent loss or weakening of pulse below insertion site • Irregular waveform on monitor screen or printout	• Trauma to vessel during catheter insertion • Artery irritated by catheter after insertion	• Notify the doctor. • Prepare lidocaine, which the doctor may inject directly into the arterial catheter to relieve the spasm. *Caution:* Make sure that the lidocaine doesn't contain epinephrine, which could cause further arterial constriction. • Document the complication as well as your interventions.	• Tape the catheter securely to prevent it from moving in the artery. • Splint the patient's limb to stabilize the catheter.
Hematoma • Swelling at insertion site and generalized swelling of limb holding the arterial line • Bleeding at site	• Blood leakage around the catheter (resulting from weakened or damaged artery) • Failure to maintain pressure at site after removing catheter	• Stop the bleeding. • If the hematoma appears while the catheter is in place, notify the doctor. • If the hematoma appears within 30 minutes after you remove the catheter, apply ice to the site. Otherwise, apply warm, moist compresses to help speed the hematoma's absorption. • Document the complication and record your interventions.	• Tape the catheter securely and splint the insertion area to prevent damage to the artery. • After the catheter is removed, apply firm, manual pressure over the site for about 10 minutes or until bleeding stops. Then apply a pressure bandage.
Inaccurate pressure readings • Patient's clinical appearance inconsistent with pressure values	*False-high values* • Transducer positioned too low • Small air bubbles in arterial line *False-low values* • Transducer positioned too high • Large air bubble in arterial line	• Relevel and rezero the transducer system. • Remove air bubbles. • Relevel and rezero the transducer system. • Remove air bubble. • Document the complication and record your interventions.	• Be sure to zero and calibrate the transducer system precisely. • Properly level the transducer at the level of the patient's right atrium (the phlebostatic axis). • Keep air from entering the pressure tubing or system. • Check the arterial waveform configuration for abnormalities.

What to do about a displaced arterial line

Your patient is in danger of hypovolemic shock from blood loss if his arterial line is pulled out or otherwise displaced. Follow these steps to avert serious complications.

What to do first
• Immediately apply direct pressure at the insertion site, and have someone summon the doctor. Because arterial blood flows under high intravascular pressure, be certain to maintain firm, direct pressure for 5 to 10 minutes to encourage clot formation at the insertion site.
• Check the patient's I.V. line and, if ordered, increase the flow rate temporarily to compensate for blood loss.

After the bleeding stops
• Apply a sterile pressure dressing.
• Reassess the patient's level of consciousness (LOC) and orientation, and offer reassurance.
• Estimate the amount of blood loss from your observations of the blood and from the changes in the patient's blood pressure and heart rate.
• Assist the doctor as he reinserts the catheter. Ensure that the patient's arm is immobilized and that the tubing and catheter are secure.
• Withdraw blood for a complete blood count and arterial blood gas analysis, as ordered.

Ongoing care
• Frequently assess the patient's vital signs, LOC, skin color and temperature, and circulation at the insertion site and beyond.
• Watch for further bleeding or hematoma formation at the insertion site.
• Once the patient's condition stabilizes, reduce the I.V. flow rate to the previous keep-vein-open level.

Removing an Arterial Line

As a nurse, you're usually responsible for removing an arterial catheter and applying a dressing. Both procedures require sterile technique. After you remove the catheter, keep pressure on the site until bleeding stops completely—otherwise, hemorrhage could result. Then, before applying the pressure dressing, inspect the site again to ensure against recurrent bleeding.

To begin, you'll need sterile gloves (two pairs); a sterile suture set; 3″ × 3″ or 4″ × 4″ sterile gauze pads; and 2″ nonallergenic tape or a large, cloth adhesive bandage.

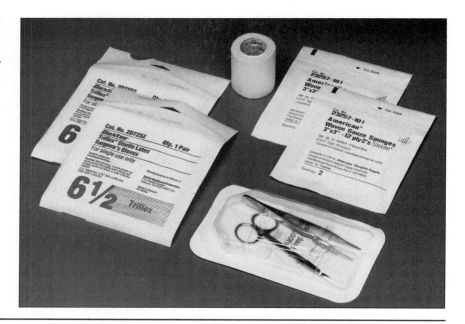

Explain the procedure to the patient. Turn off the arterial line monitor alarms but not the electrocardiogram monitor or other alarms.

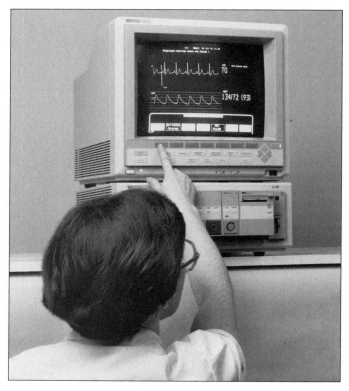

Put on the first pair of gloves. Turn the stopcock closest to the patient to the off position.

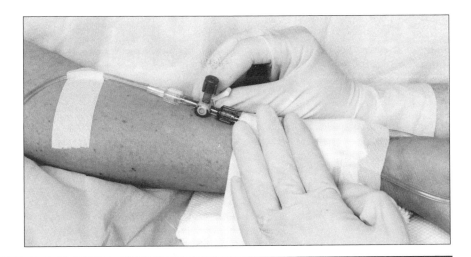

Remove the dressing, and cut and remove the sutures.

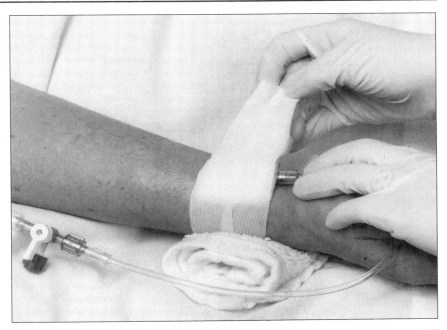

After removing the sutures, gently and quickly pull out the arterial catheter with one hand. At the same time, use the other hand to apply direct pressure to the insertion site with a 3″ × 3″ or 4″ × 4″ sterile gauze pad.

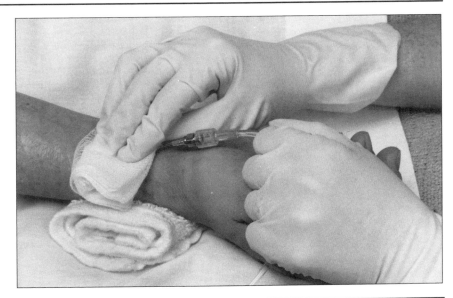

Press firmly on the site for 5 to 10 minutes or until the bleeding stops. If bleeding persists for longer than 15 minutes, notify the doctor.

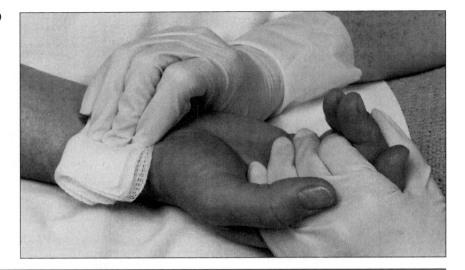

Once the bleeding stops, put on a new pair of sterile gloves. Apply a small, sterile pressure dressing to the site. Be sure to place the tape no more than three quarters of the way around the arm (as shown). Assess perfusion at the insertion site and beyond, as well as the dressing's integrity. Then dispose of the equipment according to hospital policy, and document the procedure.

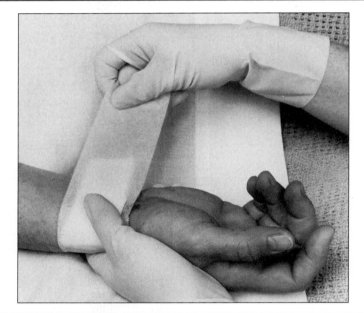

Place the patient's arm above the bed covers (as shown), and instruct the patient to keep the site above the bed covers and in clear view for at least 1 hour to ensure prompt detection of bleeding. Check the site frequently for bleeding, which may recur if the seal over the puncture site breaks.

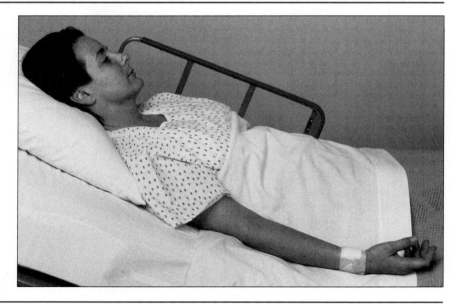

LEARNING ABOUT PULMONARY ARTERY CATHETERIZATION

Pulmonary artery catheterization can help you learn about a patient's cardiovascular and pulmonary status, obtain blood samples, and infuse solutions. With a basic pulmonary artery catheter, you can measure intracardiac pressure, pulmonary artery pressure (PAP), and cardiac output. This kind of catheter has two lumens, a balloon-inflation valve, and a thermistor.

The *distal lumen* opens into the pulmonary artery. When attached to a transducer, it allows you to measure pulmonary artery wedge pressure (PAWP) — also called pulmonary capillary wedge pressure or, sometimes, pulmonary artery obstructive pressure. The distal lumen hub is usually yellow or marked PA DISTAL.

The *proximal lumen* opens into the right atrium or the vena cava, depending on the size of the patient's heart. This lumen measures the pressure in the right atrium. It also delivers the bolus of injectate used to measure cardiac output and functions as a route for fluid infusion. The hub is usually blue or marked INJECTATE or PROXIMAL.

The *balloon-inflation valve* functions as the access point for inflating the balloon at the distal tip of the catheter for PAWP measurement.

The *thermistor*, which lies about 4 cm from the distal tip of the catheter, measures core body temperature. When connected to a cardiac output monitor, the thermistor measures temperature changes related to cardiac output.

With more sophisticated multilumen catheters, you can continuously monitor mixed venous oxygen saturation levels, intermittently measure the right ventricular volume and ejection fractions, and initiate atrial, ventricular, or atrioventricular sequential pacings.

Inserted by the doctor in the internal jugular, subclavian, femoral, or brachial vein, the catheter has a balloon tip and is flow directed, allowing venous circulation to carry it through the right atrium and ventricle to the pulmonary artery. (See *Insertion sites for a pulmonary artery catheter.*) To evaluate catheter placement, you'll set up a monitoring system and evaluate the waveforms.

Insertion sites for a pulmonary artery catheter

The most common sites for percutaneous insertion of a pulmonary artery catheter are the right internal jugular, the subclavian, and the femoral veins. The doctor may also insert a pulmonary artery catheter into the brachial vein, but this approach requires incising the vein in a cutdown procedure.

The right internal jugular is considered the safest insertion site. Although the subclavian vein is easily accessed, its use carries certain risks. The most significant risk is pneumothorax, resulting from puncturing the lung at a level above the clavicle during catheter insertion. Additionally, using the subclavian vein may cause the catheter or the introducer to bend or kink during insertion.

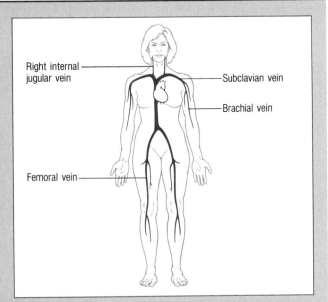

Jan M. Headley, RN, BS, who contributed to this section, is a senior education consultant with Baxter Healthcare Corp., Edwards Critical-Care Division, Irvine, Calif. The publisher thanks the following organizations for their help: Baxter Healthcare Corp., Irvine, Calif.; Doylestown (Pa.) Hospital; Dynatech Nevada Inc., Carson City, Nev.; Hewlett-Packard Co., Waltham, Mass.; and Hill-Rom, Batesville, Ind.

PREPARING FOR CATHETER INSERTION

Begin by checking the doctor's order, which indicates why the patient needs catheterization. This information will help you select the appropriate catheter, such as the basic thermodilution pulmonary artery catheter. Choose a catheter of the proper size (for most adults, a #7.5 French). Next, make sure that the sterilization date on the catheter package hasn't expired. If the doctor will insert the catheter percutaneously, you'll also need to obtain an introducer.

▶ *Clinical tip:* Check the manufacturer's recommendations when choosing an introducer. Typically, it will be a half size larger than the catheter. This guards against damaging the balloon tip during insertion. However, if you expect to infuse a large volume of fluid through the catheter's side port, select an introducer that's a full size larger than the catheter. The additional space between the catheter and introducer allows for easier fluid infusion.

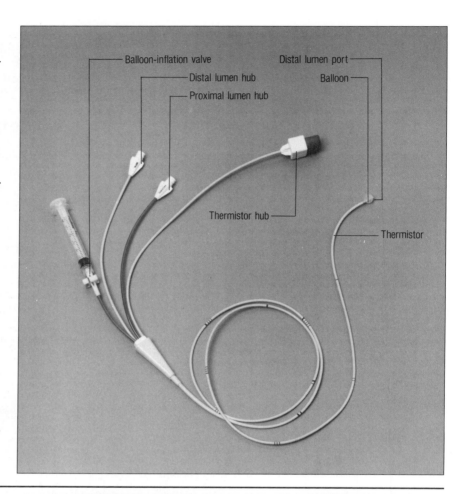

You'll also need a sterile introducer kit that contains a sterile contamination sheath. In addition, gather a sterile basin, sterile water or 0.9% sodium chloride solution, sterile and clean gloves, a face shield (or eye goggles and mask), one or more sterile gowns (depending on hospital policy), sterile drapes, povidone-iodine swabs, sutures, povidone-iodine ointment, sterile 3″ × 3″ and 4″ × 4″ gauze pads, hypoallergenic tape, a marking pen, a carpenter's level or ruler, a clean towel (optional), and lidocaine (optional).

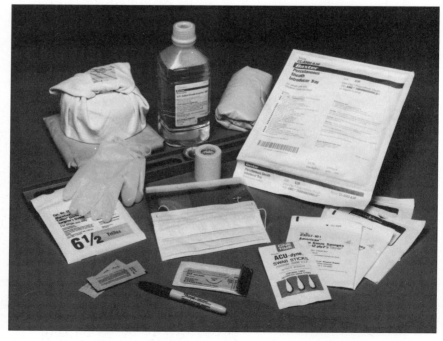

After you assemble the equipment for placing the catheter, set up the system for monitoring arterial pressures once the catheter is inserted. To monitor pulmonary artery and intermittent right atrial pressures, you'll need at least one pressure transducer and flush system (as shown). However, to continuously monitor right atrial pressure (or central venous pressure), add a second transducer and flush system to the original setup. If you think you'll need an extra pair of clean gloves, obtain them now.

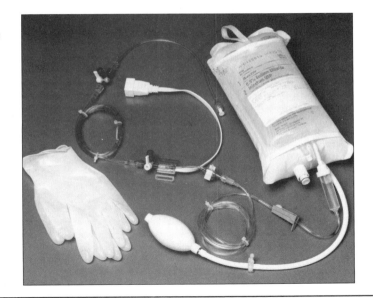

Place the crash cart close to the patient's bed in case of an emergency.

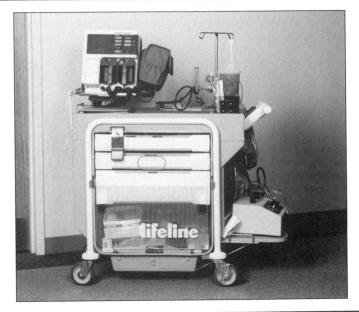

Turn on the patient's bedside monitor to give it time to warm up enough to display the waveforms accurately. (Check the manufacturer's instructions; some monitors require up to 20 minutes.) Also make sure that the monitor has the number of pressure modules needed to monitor the pressures required.

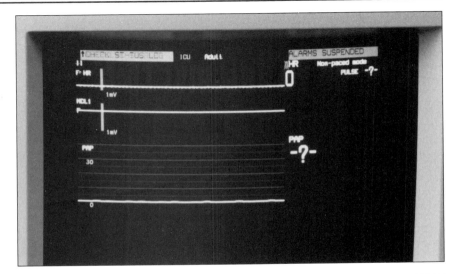

Explain the procedure to the patient and his family, and check that the patient has given informed consent for the procedure. Then take the patient's vital signs and assess cardiac rhythm.

Caution: Although pulmonary artery catheter insertion has no contraindications, patients who have a left bundle-branch block risk developing a right bundle-branch block. In such a situation, be prepared to assist with emergency pacing.

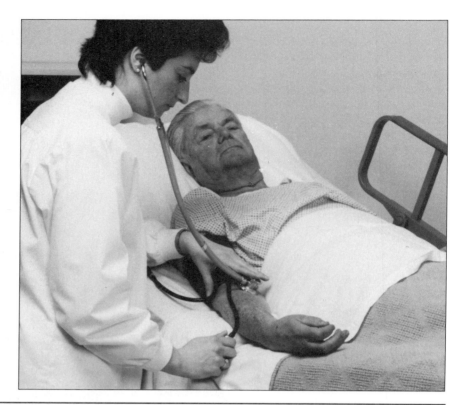

Before catheter insertion, ensure accurate pressure readings by positioning the transducer at the phlebostatic axis—the patient's fourth intercostal space and the midpoint between the anterior and posterior chest wall. (Because PAPs indirectly reflect left atrial pressures, the zero point should be level with the left atrium.) Position the transducer's air-fluid interface (located at the vent, or zero, port of the transducer's stopcock) level with this point (as shown). The head of the patient's bed may be flat or elevated.

▶ *Clinical tip:* Take care to position the transducer precisely. If the vent port is too low, pressure readings will be falsely elevated. Conversely, if the vent port is too high, pressure readings will be falsely low.

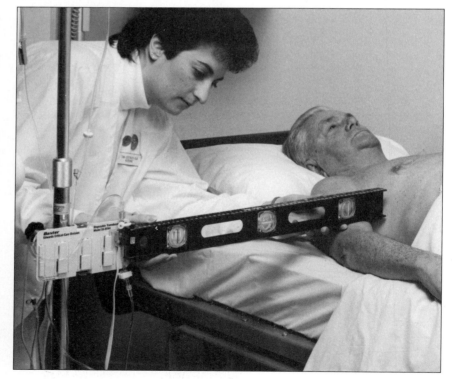

Put a piece of tape on the patient's chest, and use a marking pen to pinpoint the phlebostatic axis on the tape or the patient's chest. This marking allows every nurse to use the same reference point when obtaining pressure readings.

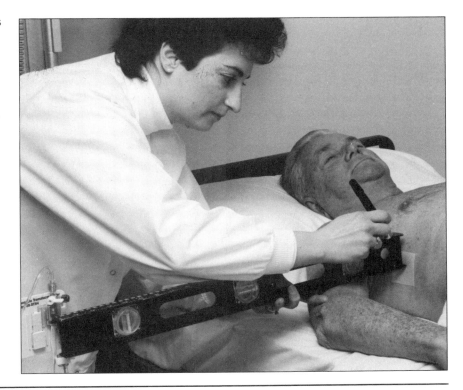

Next, remove the cap from the vent port. Then turn the stopcock off to the patient, thereby opening the transducer to air.

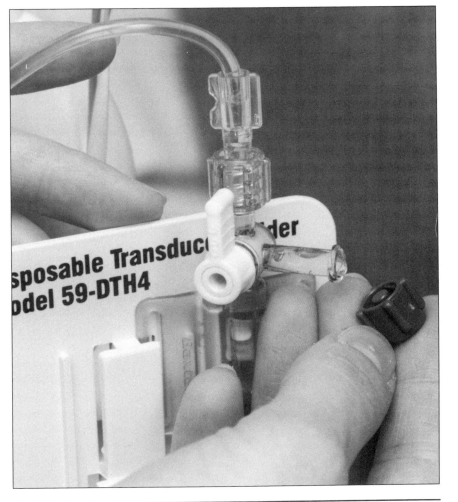

Press the ZERO button on the monitor. Then press the CALIBRATE button according to the directions supplied by the manufacturer. Keep in mind that some monitors require manipulation of a calibration button or knob and some monitors calibrate automatically.

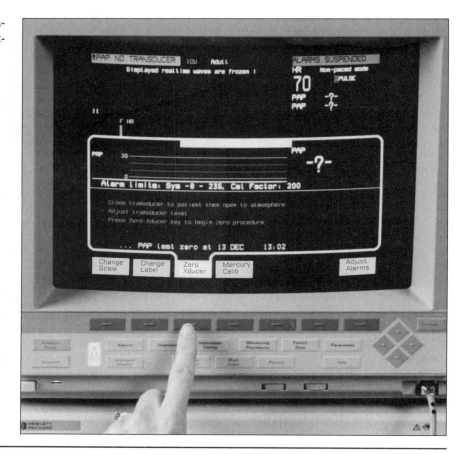

Following the manufacturer's instructions, select the appropriate mode and scale—for example, a mean pressure mode and a scale of 0 to 30 or 0 to 60 mm Hg. Keep in mind that larger scales may produce small waveforms that are difficult to read.

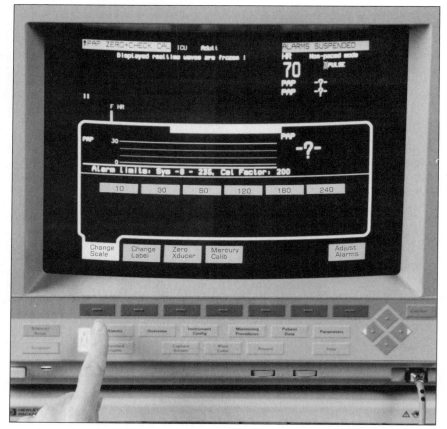

ASSISTING WITH CATHETER INSERTION

Roll an overbed table to the same side of the bed as the insertion site. Use this area to create a sterile field. Bring all of the equipment you assembled for insertion to this area.

Note: Insertion procedures may remain constant even with different insertion sites. The following steps focus on insertion through the subclavian vein.

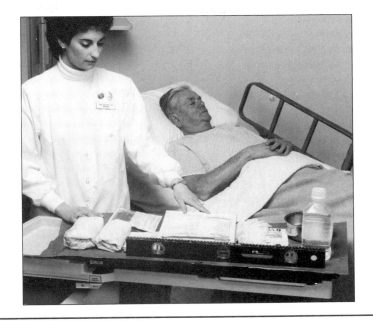

Have the patient lie on his back without a pillow. Adjust the bed to the desired height, and place the patient in a slight Trendelenburg's position. If necessary to help the doctor locate the insertion site, place a rolled towel under the patient's scapula.

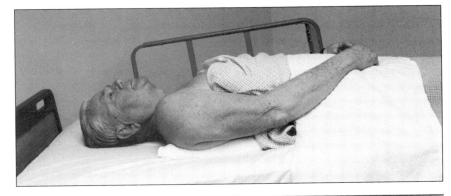

While the doctor puts on a face shield (or goggles and mask), sterile gown, and sterile gloves, you'll need to put on a face shield (or goggles and mask), a gown, and clean gloves. Throughout the procedure, observe universal precautions.

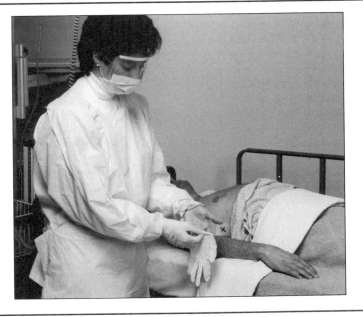

As the doctor cleans the insertion site with povidone-iodine swabs (or ointment) and drapes the insertion area, position the patient's face away from the insertion site. This keeps the patient from breathing on and contaminating the site. It also facilitates insertion of the catheter.

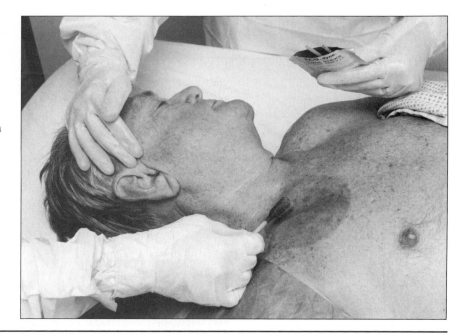

Maintaining sterile technique, assist with opening the prepackaged introducer and with its insertion. Continuing to maintain sterile technique, open the outer wrapping of the pulmonary artery catheter, positioning it so that the doctor can remove the inner sterile package. After the doctor opens the inner wrapping, prepares the catheter insertion tray, and applies the contamination sheath, he'll hand you the lumen hubs. Be sure to touch only the hubs of the catheter.

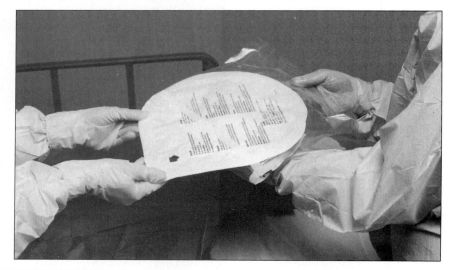

Continuing to use sterile technique, connect the pressure tubing to the distal catheter lumens. Using the pressure tubing fast-flush device, flush the lumen. (You may use a syringe containing sterile heparinized flush solution or a sterile I.V. setup to flush the proximal lumen before connecting the pressure tubing.)

Note: If you're using multiple-pressure lines, make sure that the distal lumen is attached to the line that will reflect pressure on the monitor screen. If it isn't, you won't obtain the correct waveform.

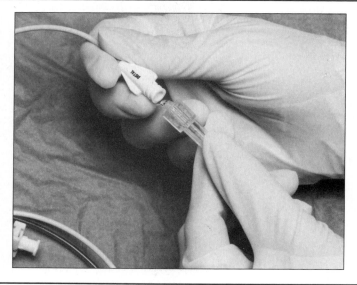

Before inserting the catheter, the doctor will inflate the balloon with air to ensure its integrity. Inspect the inflated balloon for symmetrical shape. Pour sterile water or 0.9% sodium chloride solution into a small sterile basin so that the doctor can submerge the balloon to check for bubbles indicating a leak.

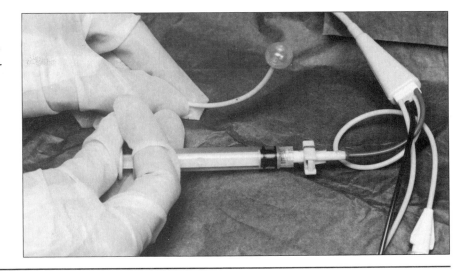

After deflating the balloon, the doctor will insert the catheter through the introducer and gently advance the catheter 15 to 20 cm to a point marked on the catheter by two black bands. At this distance, the catheter should have exited the end of the introducer sheath and be near the junction of the superior vena cava and right atrium. The monitor should display oscillations consistent with the patient's respirations. If the patient is awake, have him cough or take some deep breaths to enhance the oscillations.

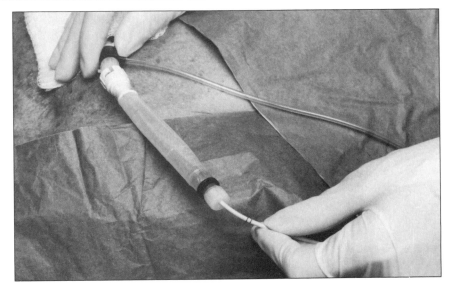

As ordered, use the volume-limited 3-cc syringe in the pulmonary artery catheter package to inflate the balloon. Verify the maximum balloon inflation volume printed on the shaft of the catheter. Typically, you'll use 1.5 cc of air for a #7.5 French catheter. Avoid overinflating the balloon, which causes the balloon to lose elasticity or to rupture.

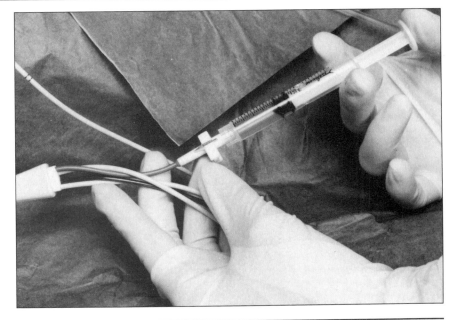

To keep the balloon inflated, close the red gate valve (or the appropriate stopcock) on the catheter (as shown).

Note: Insertion is the only time you'll use this valve or stopcock to keep the balloon inflated.

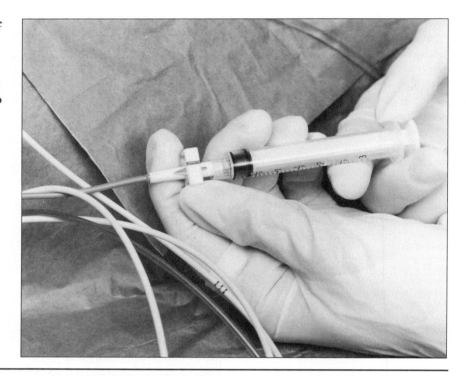

As the doctor advances the catheter, monitor waveforms, pressure values (which provide evidence of the catheter's location), and electrocardiogram tracings. If possible, obtain printed waveforms for each chamber. Watch closely for the waveform indicating that the catheter has advanced between 20 and 25 cm to the right atrium (as shown). Typically, you'll see two small waves for each PQRST complex. You should also observe a normal mean pressure ranging between 2 and 6 mm Hg.

Note: Pressure ranges cited in this section reflect standards accepted by the American Association of Critical-Care Nurses (AACN) and published in the AACN's 1991 *Core Curriculum for Critical Care Nursing.*

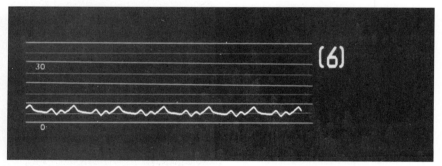

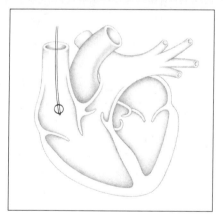

When the catheter advances 30 to 35 cm, its tip should enter the right ventricle. Watch for a right ventricular waveform, such as the one shown at right. Also keep track of pressure values. Normal systolic pressure ranges from 20 to 30 mm Hg; normal diastolic pressure, from 0 to 5 mm Hg. Pay particular attention to the diastolic pressure. An increase indicates that the catheter has advanced into the pulmonary artery.

▶ *Clinical tip:* Keep a bolus of lidocaine handy and remain alert for ventricular ectopy when the catheter enters the right ventricle. Usually, ventricular irritability subsides when the catheter tip reaches the pulmonary artery. If not, the doctor may withdraw the catheter or order lidocaine.

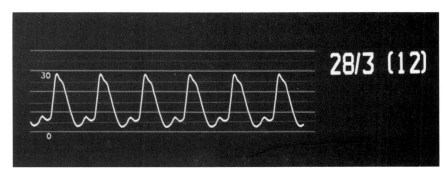

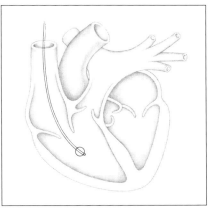

Continue watching the monitor for a waveform showing that the catheter has advanced 35 to 40 cm into the pulmonary artery. You should see a smooth upstroke (reflecting systole) and a downstroke (representing diastole) and a dicrotic notch resulting from the pulmonic valve closing. The closed valve also accounts for the higher diastolic pressure ranges. Normally, PAPs range as follows: systolic, 20 to 30 mm Hg; diastolic, 10 to 20 mm Hg; and mean, 10 to 15 mm Hg.

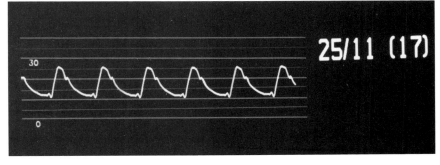

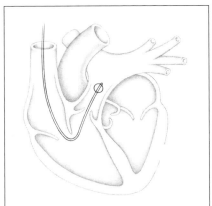

Seeing catheter markings between 40 and 50 cm at the insertion site indicates that the circulation has carried the catheter tip to a distal branch of the pulmonary artery. Now, you can assess the PAWP, derived from the inflated balloon wedged in this area. Because the balloon occludes blood flow from the pulmonary artery and the right side of the heart, the waveform and pressure values reflect pressure in the left atrium. At this point, the normal mean pressure ranges between 6 and 12 mm Hg.

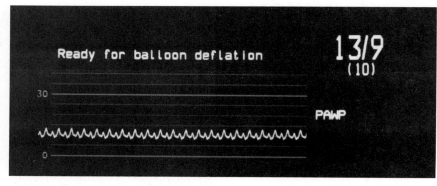

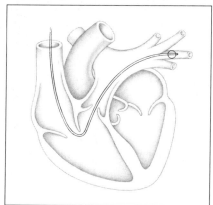

After noting this pressure, unlock the gate valve and detach the syringe. This allows the balloon to deflate passively. Never aspirate air to deflate the balloon. Doing so could cause the balloon to lose elasticity.

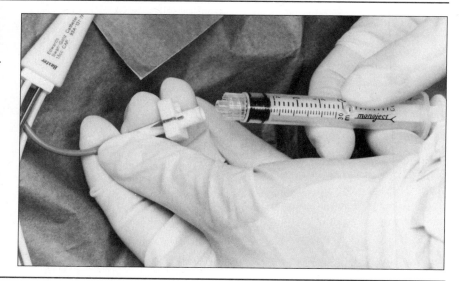

To ensure that the balloon has deflated, observe the monitor for the return of the PAP waveform (as shown).

Caution: Leaving the balloon inflated for a prolonged time could result in a pulmonary infarction.

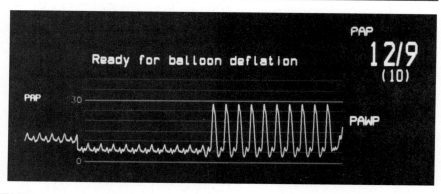

Next, the doctor will withdraw the catheter between 1 and 2 cm to remove any loop that may have formed in the right ventricle, decreasing the chance for catheter migration.

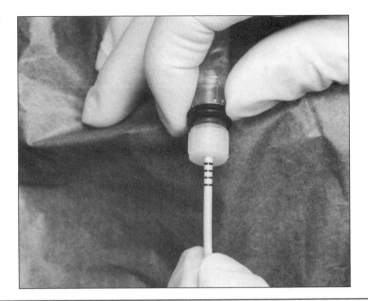

Slowly reinflate the balloon until you again obtain a PAWP wave-form. Note the amount of air required to obtain the tracing; it should still be 1.5 cc.

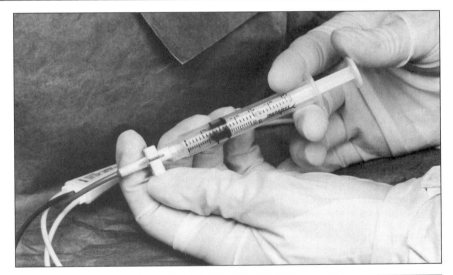

Once you're sure that the catheter is properly positioned, remove the syringe and allow the balloon to deflate passively. Again check the monitor for resumption of the PAP waveform. If the doctor hasn't already sutured the introducer in place, he usually does so now.

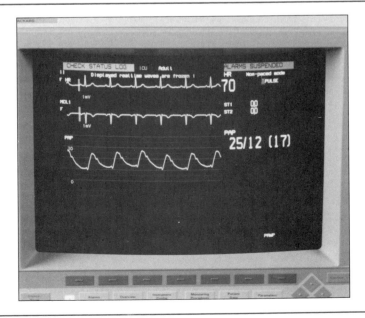

Take off your clean gloves, and put on sterile gloves to apply a sterile, occlusive dressing over the insertion site. Arrange for a bedside chest X-ray to verify correct catheter placement.

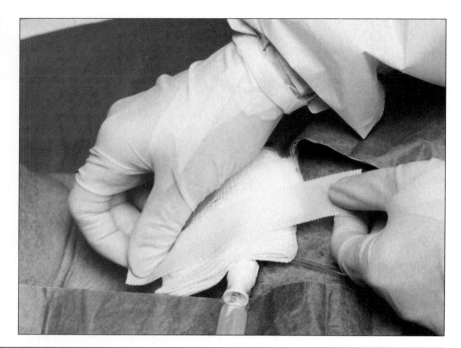

Document the procedure, noting the date and time, the insertion site, the doctor who inserted the catheter, the type of dressing applied, the concentration of the heparinized flush solution, and the patient's tolerance of the procedure. Also document the pressures and waveforms obtained for each heart chamber during insertion. Record whether any arrhythmias occurred during or after insertion, and note the volume of air required to obtain a PAWP tracing.

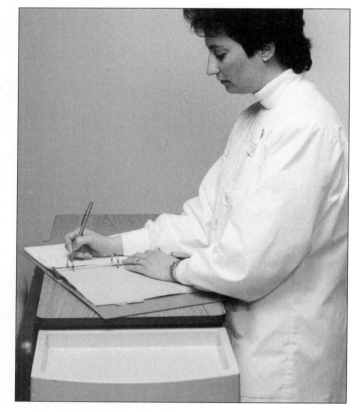

MANAGING A PULMONARY ARTERY LINE

When your patient has a pulmonary artery line, your responsibilities include caring for the catheter insertion site and the catheter as well as monitoring pulmonary artery pressure (PAP), right atrial pressure (RAP), and pulmonary artery wedge pressure (PAWP).

You'll change the dressing according to hospital policy (usually every 24 hours), observe the site for infection and catheter slippage or kinking, and document these procedures.

How often you'll need to obtain pressure readings will vary with the patient's condition. For example, routine orders may require you to note PAP and PAWP every 1 to 4 hours. If the patient's condition is unstable or if you need to evaluate certain treatment effects, you'll take readings more often. However, you'll need to limit the frequency of PAWP measurements in patients who are elderly, who have pulmonary hypertension, or who are otherwise at high risk for pulmonary artery rupture.

Pulmonary artery rupture is a rare but life-threatening risk for any patient undergoing PAWP measurement. That's why some hospitals allow only doctors or specially trained nurses to perform the procedure.

Measuring PAP and other pressures

PAP, RAP, and PAWP are the pressures you'll measure. To monitor PAP, place the patient in a supine position (as shown). If he can't tolerate being completely flat, raise the head of the bed slightly. Then level, zero, and balance the transducer system, as described in "Assisting with catheter insertion" earlier in this section.

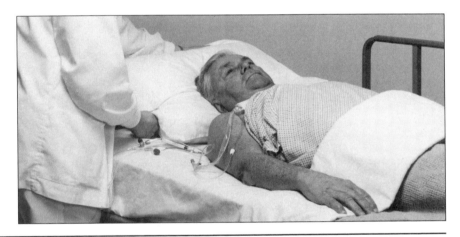

Note and record the systolic and diastolic PAP values. To obtain an accurate PAP reading, record the value at end-expiration in the respiratory cycle. *Never* remove the patient from a ventilator to obtain a measurement. If rapid or irregular respirations interfere with identifying the end-expiration period, average the measurements through an entire respiratory cycle.

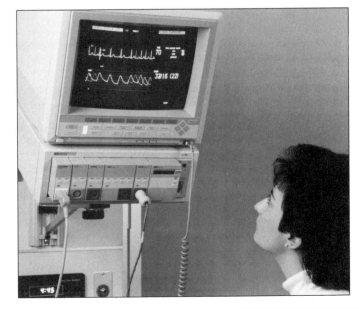

If the patient's monitoring system continuously measures PAP and only intermittently measures RAP, turn the stopcock on the transducer in the appropriate direction: off to the distal lumen for PAP and on to the proximal lumen for RAP.

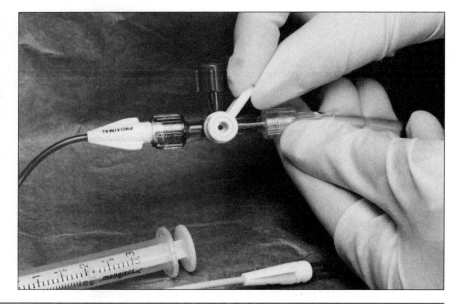

Check the monitor to observe the waveform change from PAP to RAP (as shown). Record the measured pressure. Then return the stopcock to the position for PAP. Recheck the monitor to make sure that it again displays the PAP waveform.

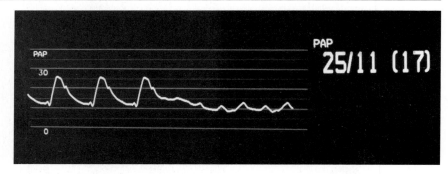

If you're continuously monitoring the patient's RAP, observe the monitor screen for the RAP value. Then record your findings.

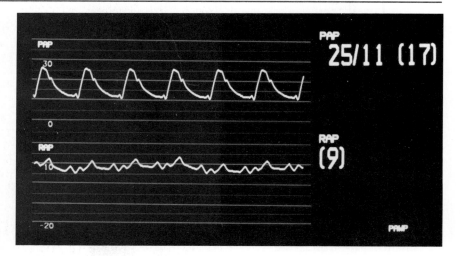

To obtain the PAWP value, first adjust the monitor to the mean mode. Then check the transducer to ensure that it's still properly leveled. Your next step will be to wedge the catheter in a more distal branch of the pulmonary artery to help evaluate left ventricular pressure and function. To do so, remove the volume-limited syringe from the balloon-inflation valve that comes with the pulmonary artery catheter.

Note: Gloves are optional, depending on the situation.

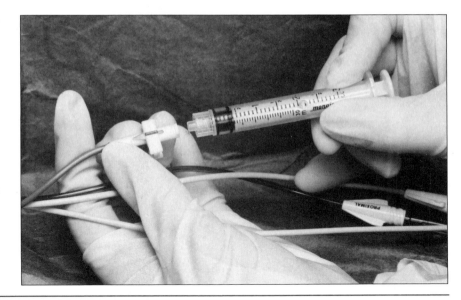

Pull back the plunger of the syringe until it stops, which should be at 1.5 cc.

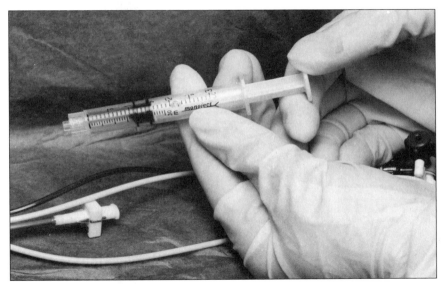

Reattach the syringe to the balloon-inflation valve.

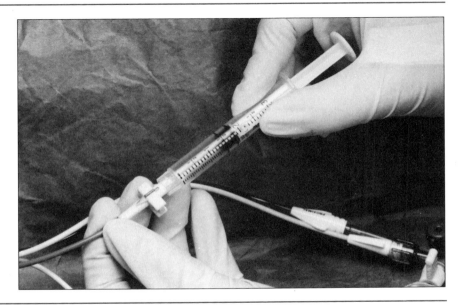

Slowly depress the plunger to inflate the balloon. You should feel *slight* resistance. If you feel marked resistance or no resistance at all, stop inflating the balloon immediately.

Caution: Lack of resistance suggests a ruptured balloon.

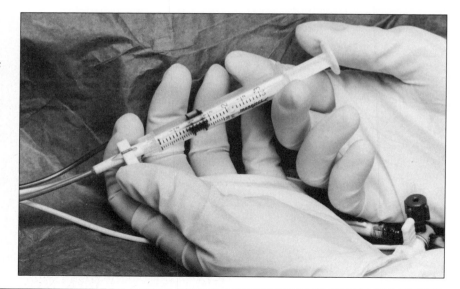

As you inflate the balloon, look for a PAWP waveform on the monitor (as shown). As soon as this tracing pattern appears, stop inflating the balloon. Never inject more air than the minimum required to obtain a wedge tracing, and never inject more than 1.5 cc. Quickly read the pressure.

▶ *Clinical tip:* Keep careful track of the pressure needed to inflate the balloon. If a wedge tracing appears after injecting less than 1.25 cc of air, then the catheter has migrated to a more distal portion of the pulmonary artery.

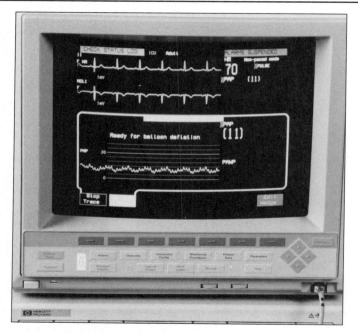

Next, detach the syringe from the pulmonary artery catheter so that the balloon deflates passively. Never leave the balloon inflated over more than two respiratory cycles, or 10 to 15 seconds. Doing so could induce a pulmonary infarction.

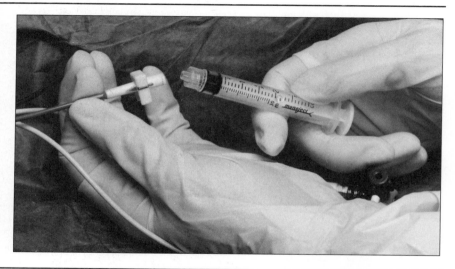

Maintaining a pulmonary artery catheter

Ensure that the patient's bedside monitor continuously displays the PAP waveform. This way, you'll immediately recognize waveform changes signifying problems with the pulmonary artery catheter, such as a migrating tip that lodges, rather than floats, in the vessel. Arrange for daily chest X-rays, as ordered, to verify proper catheter placement.

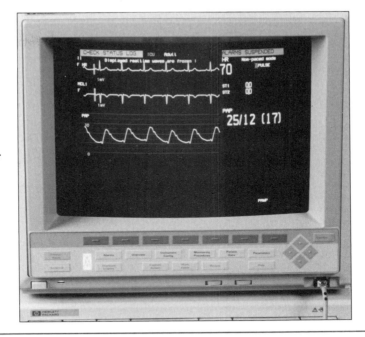

Ensure a constant flush rate of 3 ml/hour. To do this, continuously monitor the pressure bag portion of the flush system (as shown). This apparatus should stay inflated at 300 mm Hg—the pressure needed to maintain the flush rate.

▶ *Clinical tip:* Always watch the PAP waveform. As long as you see a clear waveform with clear dicrotic notches, you won't need to flush the system manually. Also make sure that the flush solution is the only agent infused through the distal port. Don't use this port for any other fluids or drugs.

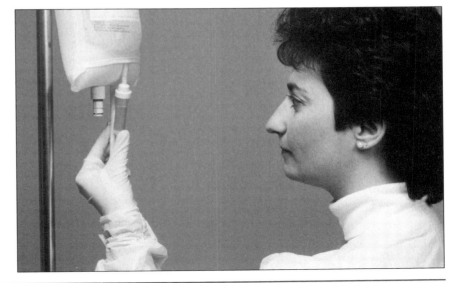

Then check the right atrial (RA) lumen. If you're monitoring RAP— either continuously or intermittently—this lumen should have a flush system attached (as shown) to keep it patent. If you're using the RA lumen only for instilling injectate to assess cardiac output, you can maintain patency with an I.V. drip. In such a case, make sure that the solution infuses at a minimum rate of 10 ml/hour.

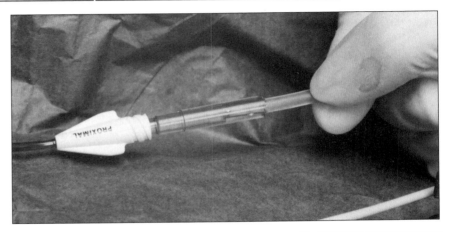

Responding to abnormal waveforms and pressures

When your patient has a pulmonary artery catheter, do you know how to respond to an uncharacteristic waveform on the monitor? For example, what action should you take for an erratic waveform? How should you respond to a concurrent arrhythmia on the electrocardiogram (ECG)? How can you deal with an obviously inaccurate pressure reading? Use the following to help you recognize and resolve common problems.

No waveform on monitor
A waveform may fail to appear on the monitor for several reasons—for example, the transducer is not open to the catheter, the transducer or monitor has been set up improperly, or a catheter is clotted.

Corrective measures include checking the stopcock, calibration, or scale mechanisms; tightening connections; rezeroing the setup; or replacing the transducer.

Overdamped waveform
If air bubbles, blood clots, or a catheter tip lodged in the vessel wall causes an overdamped waveform to appear on the patient's monitor, you may correct the problem in several ways.

Try removing any air bubbles observed in the catheter tubing and transducer. Try restoring patency to a clotted catheter by aspirating the clot with a syringe. (*Never* irrigate the line as a first step.) Or try moving a lodged catheter by repositioning the patient or by having him cough and breathe deeply. If you need to move the catheter itself, do so only according to hospital policy.

Changed waveform configuration
Noisy or erratic tracings may result from an incorrectly positioned catheter, loose connections in the setup, or faulty electrical circuitry.

Respond to this problem by repositioning the patient (or the catheter, if necessary), arranging for a chest X-ray to verify catheter location, or checking and tightening connections in the catheter and transducer apparatus.

Catheter fling
An erratic waveform may also result from catheter fling, which reflects excessive catheter movement (possibly caused by an arrhythmia or excessive respiratory effort). In such a case, you may need to reposition the catheter according to hospital policy.

False pressure readings
If the monitor records pressures that are inaccurately too high or too low, try repositioning the transducer (level with the phlebostatic axis) or rezeroing the monitor setup.

Ventricular irritability
An ECG tracing indicating an arrhythmia may result from the catheter irritating the ventricular endocardium or the heart valves.

After confirming this arrhythmia on the patient's ECG, notify the doctor and administer antiarrhythmic drugs, as ordered.

Note: The doctor may prevent this problem during insertion by keeping the balloon inflated when advancing the catheter through the heart.

Right ventricular waveform
A pulmonary artery catheter migrating into the right ventricle will produce a ventricular tracing.

In this situation, inflate the balloon with 1.5 cc of air to move the catheter back to the pulmonary artery. If this measure fails, notify the doctor immediately so that he can reposition the catheter.

Continuous PAWP waveform
In obtaining the pulmonary artery wedge pressure (PAWP) to evaluate ventricular function, the catheter may migrate or the balloon may remain inflated. Either situation may cause a continuous PAWP waveform to appear.

To correct this, reposition the patient or have him cough and breathe deeply. Keep the balloon inflated no longer than two respiratory cycles or 15 seconds.

Missing PAWP waveform
The monitor may fail to record a PAWP waveform—possibly from a malpositioned catheter, insufficient air in the balloon tip, or even a ruptured balloon.

To intervene:
• reposition the patient (don't aspirate the balloon)
• reinflate the balloon adequately (remove the syringe from the balloon lumen, wait for the balloon to deflate passively, and then instill the correct volume of air)
• assess the balloon's competence (note resistance during inflation, feel how the syringe's plunger springs back after the balloon inflates, and check for blood leaking from the balloon lumen).

If the balloon has ruptured, turn the patient onto his left side, tape the balloon-inflation port, and notify the doctor.

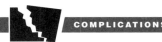

COMPLICATIONS

Dealing with hazards of pulmonary artery lines

Any patient who has a pulmonary artery catheter in place is at risk for several complications. Besides observing the patient's electrocardiogram, waveform pattern, and pressure values on the bedside monitor, watch for the following signs and symptoms of complications. Implement appropriate care measures to resolve or prevent them. Keep in mind that these procedures vary according to each state's nurse practice act.

Bacteremia
If your patient has an elevated temperature, chills, warm skin, headache, and malaise, he's showing signs and symptoms of an infection, such as bacteremia. Administer antibiotic medications as ordered. To prevent such an infection, maintain sterile technique. Also be sure to maintain and change the monitoring setup according to hospital policy.

Bleedback
Caused by leaks in the pulmonary artery catheter apparatus or a pressure bag that's inflated below 300 mm Hg, bleedback is easily seen in the pressure tubing. To intervene early, be sure to tighten connections in the monitoring setup. Preventive measures include returning stopcocks to their proper position after use and keeping the pressure bag adequately inflated.

Bleeding at the insertion site
If the patient has prolonged oozing or frank bleeding at the insertion site after catheter withdrawal, apply firm pressure until the bleeding stops. To prevent this problem, maintain pressure on the site during catheter withdrawal and for at least 10 minutes afterward, and apply a pressure dressing over the site. At a femoral site, apply a sandbag for 1 to 2 hours. (Also be sure to assess distal circulation routinely to ensure that a hematoma isn't obstructing blood flow.)

Pulmonary embolism
A thrombus that migrates from the catheter into pulmonary circulation or a catheter tip clotted from inadequate flushing may cause a pulmonary embolism. To prevent this, administer anticoagulants as ordered, and use a continuous flush system.

If prevention fails and your patient shows signs and symptoms of pulmonary embolism, such as sharp and stabbing chest pain, anxiety, cyanosis, dyspnea, tachypnea, and diaphoresis, try to aspirate blood (don't irrigate if you suspect an embolus). If you can't aspirate blood, a pulmonary embolus may be obstructing the line. Notify the doctor at once.

Ruptured pulmonary artery
In pulmonary artery rupture (from pulmonary hypertension, thrombus, catheter migration into the peripheral branch of the artery, or improper inflation or prolonged wedging of the catheter's balloon), the patient will experience restlessness, tachycardia, hypotension, hemoptysis, and dyspnea. In such a situation, notify the doctor immediately.

Keep in mind several preventive measures:
• Slowly inflate the balloon only until the PAWP waveform appears on the monitor, and then let the balloon deflate passively.
• Never overinflate the balloon.
• Reposition a migrating catheter (if permitted).

Pulmonary infarction
Chest pain, hemoptysis, fever, pleural friction rub, and low arterial oxygen levels point to pulmonary infarction, possibly from the catheter migrating into a wedged position in the blood vessel. Don't flush the catheter if you suspect that it has migrated. Do monitor pulmonary artery pressure continuously and notify the doctor.

Never allow the balloon to be inflated for more than two respiratory cycles or 15 seconds.

REMOVING A PULMONARY ARTERY CATHETER

Typically, a pulmonary artery catheter stays in place no longer than 3 days. In most states, pulmonary artery catheter removal is not considered within the nurse's domain. In other states, advanced collaborative standards of practice allow skilled nurses to perform this procedure. Before attempting to remove a pulmonary artery catheter, however, check with your hospital administrator about practice requirements and legal responsibilities in your locality.

To remove a pulmonary artery catheter, you'll need a suture removal kit, sterile 3″ × 3″ or 4″ × 4″ gauze pads, sterile gloves, antimicrobial swabs, and hypoallergenic tape. You'll also need equipment for observing universal precautions. Gather a face shield (or goggles and mask), a gown, and gloves.

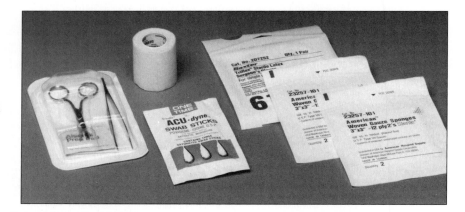

Explain the procedure to the patient as you take his vital signs and note the electrocardiogram (ECG) pattern. As ordered, obtain a chest X-ray to check for kinks or knots in the catheter.

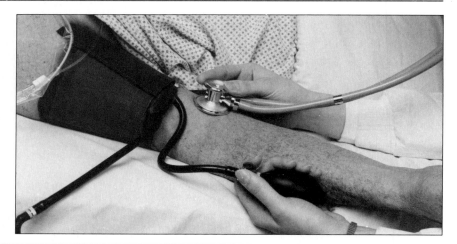

If possible, place the patient in a supine position.

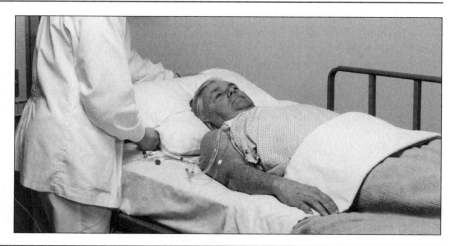

If you're removing the catheter from the subclavian or internal jugular vein, turn the patient's face away from the site.

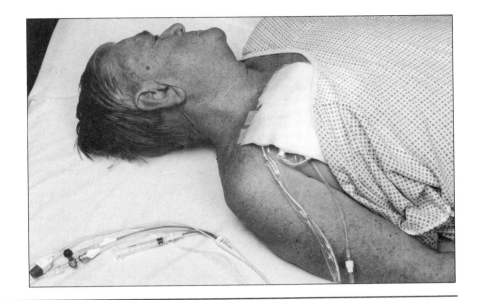

Put on gloves, gown, and face shield, and gently remove the dressing from the catheter site. Assist the doctor as he takes out the sutures. If you're removing the catheter, take out the sutures yourself. If the introducer will remain in place, leave the sutures securing the introducer intact. Then dispose of the dressing and remove your gloves.

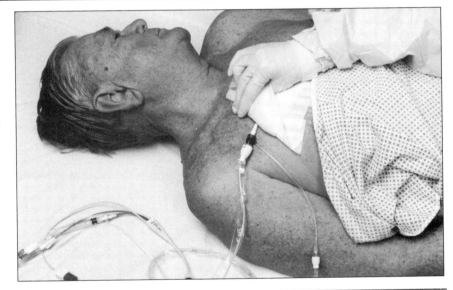

Turn all stopcocks off to the patient.

Caution: To observe the waveforms during removal, leave the stopcocks turned on to the distal port. Keep in mind that an air embolism may result, so exercise extreme caution when doing so.

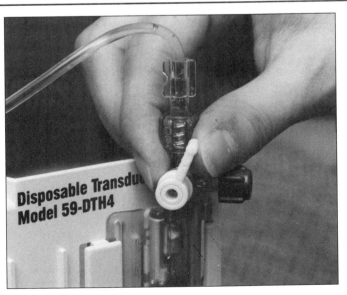

Next, make sure that the balloon is deflated.

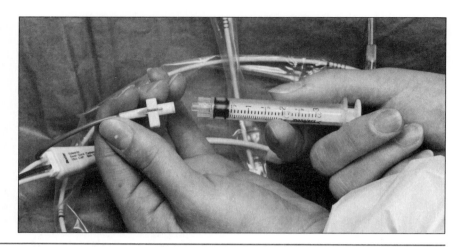

If you'll be removing the catheter, put on sterile gloves.

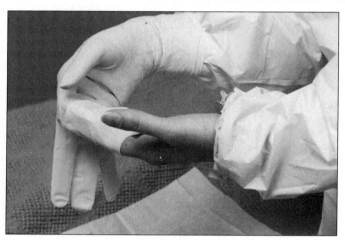

Slowly and smoothly withdraw the catheter (near right); at the same time watch the monitor for arrhythmias.

Caution: If you feel any resistance, stop immediately and notify the doctor.

If you remove both the catheter and the introducer, apply pressure to the site using the sterile gauze pads. If the introducer will remain in place, observe the introducer's diaphragm for a bleedback. If you observe no bleedback, assume that the hemostatic valve within the introducer is intact. Next, clean the site with antimicrobial swabs before covering it with a sterile occlusive dressing (far right). Then document the date and time of catheter removal and the patient's tolerance of the procedure. Include a current description of the insertion site.

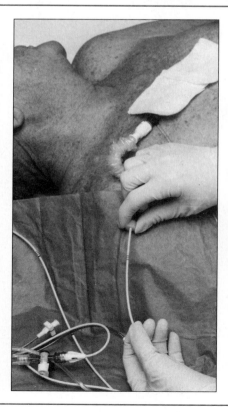

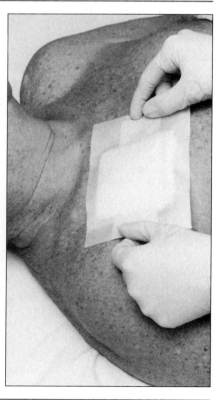

LEARNING ABOUT C.V.P. MONITORING

Central venous pressure (CVP) is monitored with either a pressure transducer system or a water manometer. Both kinds of equipment accommodate intermittent or continuous CVP monitoring. The monitor is connected to a catheter that has been threaded through the subclavian or jugular vein (or the basilic, cephalic, or saphenous veins) to a position in or near the right atrium.

In a critically ill patient, a central venous line allows you to obtain pressure readings, blood for laboratory samples, and access to a large vessel for rapid administration of large amounts of fluid.

When the left ventricle is functioning normally, CVP monitoring helps evaluate the patient's cardiac status and response to fluid administration. CVP values assist you in evaluating venous return to the heart and in indirectly determining how well the heart is pumping.

CORRELATING C.V.P. WITH CARDIAC FUNCTION

Essentially, CVP measurements reflect events in the cardiac cycle and, in so doing, depict cardiac function. During ventricular diastole, the atrioventricular (AV) valves open. As diastole ends, each open valve creates what amounts to a common heart chamber. The pressure created by blood volume in the ventricles now extends back into the atria so that pressure measured in the right atrium indirectly mirrors the volume status of the right ventricle (called preload). During systole, the AV valves close and the semilunar valves open. Now the pressure measured in the atria indicates atrial filling.

FACTORS AFFECTING C.V.P.

Anything that affects the patient's hydration status can affect CVP. For example, an increase in circulating volume is reflected as an increase in venous return to the heart and will cause CVP to rise. (See *What causes CVP changes?*)

Certain mechanical factors can also affect CVP. For example, if your patient is on a ventilator, his intrathoracic pressure will be higher on inspiration and lower on expiration—the opposite of normal respirations. When monitoring CVP in such a case, take the reading at end-expiration.

 INSIGHTS AND INTERPRETATIONS

What causes CVP changes?

Although most experts consider 3.7 to 7.4 mm Hg (5 to 10 cm H_2O) a normal range for central venous pressure (CVP), this range may vary slightly (for example, 1.5 to 5.9 mm Hg [2 to 8 cm H_2O]). The factors that may cause changes include conditions that alter venous return, circulating blood volume, or cardiac performance.

Note CVP changes that indicate a trend: The trend may be more significant than the individual values. For example, patients with chronic pulmonary problems, such as cor pulmonale, may have high CVP values without acute heart failure.

To interpret pressure readings correctly, establish the patient's baseline CVP; then measure CVP at 15-, 30-, and 60-minute intervals. Report fluctuations of more than 1.5 mm Hg (2 cm H_2O), which may indicate a change in the patient's status.

What increases CVP?
• Increased venous return from conditions that cause hypervolemic states, such as volume overload or hepatic disease
• Depressed cardiac function
• Vasoconstriction
• Cardiac tamponade
• Chronic or acute pulmonary hypertension
• Positive end-expiratory pressure administered with mechanical ventilation

What decreases CVP?
• Decreased venous return and hypovolemia from hemorrhage or dehydration
• Loss of vascular tone caused by vasodilation (for example, from sepsis), which contributes to venous pooling and reduced blood return to the heart

---

Contributors to this section are *Jan M. Headley, RN, BS,* a senior education consultant at Baxter Healthcare Corp., Edwards Critical-Care Division, Irvine, Calif.; and *Paulette Dorney, RN, MSN, CCRN,* a critical care staff development instructor at North Penn Hospital, Lansdale, Pa. The publisher thanks the following organizations for their help: *Baxter Healthcare Corp., Edwards Critical-Care Division,* Irvine, Calif.; *Hewlett-Packard Co.,* Waltham, Mass.; and *Hill-Rom,* Batesville, Ind.

MONITORING C.V.P. WITH A PRESSURE TRANSDUCER

If you're attaching the central venous catheter to a computerized pressure transducer monitoring system, such as the one described on these pages, you can use either the proximal lumen of a pulmonary artery catheter or a single-lumen central venous catheter. If the catheter has several lumens, one lumen can be used for continuous central venous pressure (CVP) monitoring and the others for fluid administration.

Although you'll care for and maintain the catheter in this system as you would any catheter, you'll obtain the pressure values in a different way. This monitoring system communicates pressure values in digital form on the monitor screen. A CVP waveform display is another feature of this system.

Gather a prepared pressure transducer setup and a carpenter's level. Take them to the patient's bedside. You'll also need tape and a marking pen.

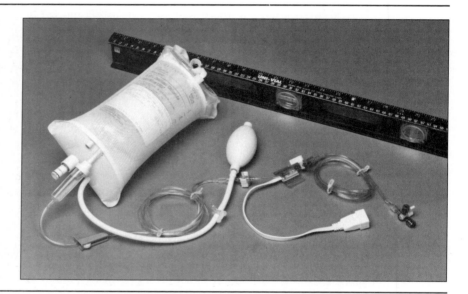

Explain the procedure to the patient, answer his questions, and reassure him. Wash your hands. Place the patient in a supine position if he can tolerate it. If not, use semi-Fowler's position. Make sure that you note the patient's position on his chart.

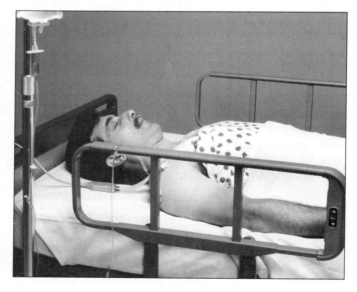

If the pressure transducer cable isn't already attached to the pressure module of the monitor, attach it now. *(Note:* If your hospital policy requires you to wear gloves or if you think leakage may occur, put on gloves.)

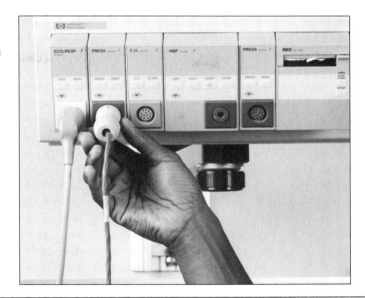

Then, if the prepared pressure transducer setup isn't attached to the appropriate lumen of the pulmonary artery catheter or the central venous catheter, attach it (as shown).

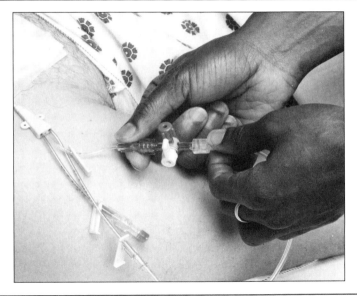

Locate the patient's phlebostatic axis by mentally bisecting the fourth intercostal space at the midpoint of the anteroposterior chest wall. (You can also use the midaxillary line, but doing so may produce less accurate pressure readings than using the midpoint landmark.) Then put a piece of tape on the patient's side, and use a marking pen to pinpoint the phlebostatic axis, which is level with the right atrium. Position the transducer level with the mark.

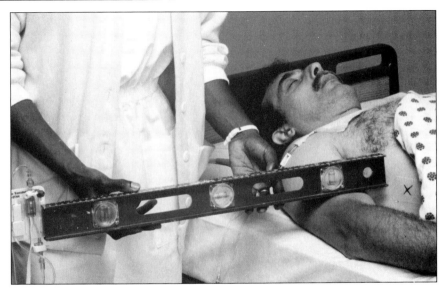

Turn the stopcock so that it's closed to the patient and open to air.

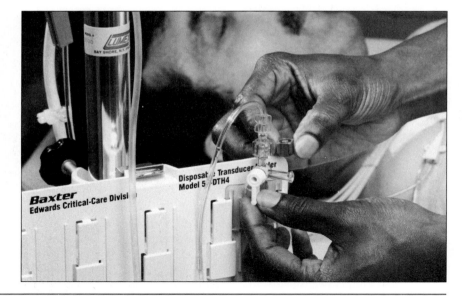

Next, zero the monitor by pressing the ZERO XDUCER key (as shown).

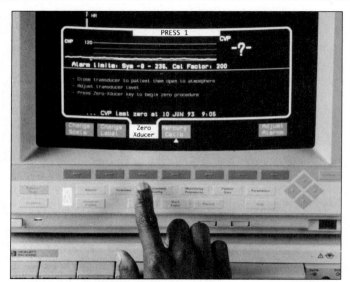

Afterward, position the stopcock so that it's closed to air and open to the patient. Then watch for CVP waveforms to appear on the monitor.

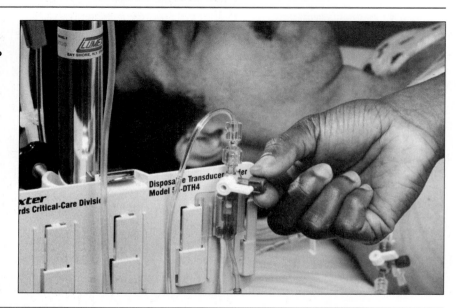

Check the monitor scale. If it's incorrect, select the proper scale by pressing the designated monitor key. (Consult the manufacturer's directions.)

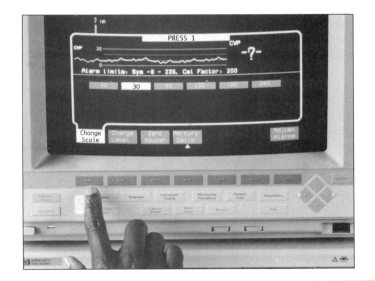

The amplitude of the CVP waveform reflects the phase of the respiratory cycle. Observe the CVP waveform for alterations resulting from unusual respiratory variations. Note the pressure value at end-expiration, and document this value on the patient's chart.

▶ *Clinical tip:* You may want to obtain a printout of the CVP tracing for reference when the waveform shows several respiratory variations.

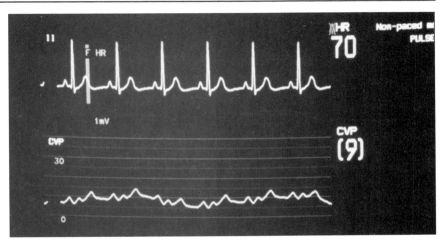

Converting pressure values

Although the water manometer—the first device developed for monitoring central venous pressure at the bedside—is still in use today, the pressure transducer system is used in most hospitals. Both methods measure right atrial pressure—the pressure transducer in millimeters of mercury (mm Hg) and the water manometer in centimeters of water (cm H_2O). If your hospital uses both pressure transducers and water manometers, you may have to convert pressure values.

Use this formula to convert cm H_2O to mm Hg:

$$cm\ H_2O \div 1.36 = mm\ Hg$$

Conversely, use this formula to change mm Hg to cm H_2O:

$$mm\ Hg \times 1.36 = cm\ H_2O$$

INSIGHTS AND INTERPRETATIONS

Understanding the CVP waveform

When the CVP catheter is attached to a pressure monitoring system, the bedside monitor can usually display digital pressure values, CVP waveforms, and electrocardiogram (ECG) tracings. Synchronizing the CVP waveform with the ECG helps you identify components of the tracing. Keep in mind that cardiac electrical activity precedes the mechanical activities of systole and diastole.

Normal waveforms

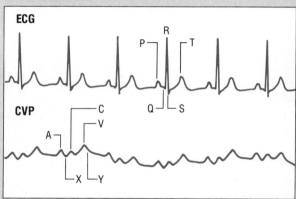

Comparing electrical activity

The P wave on the ECG reflects atrial depolarization, which is then followed by atrial contraction and increased atrial pressure. Corresponding to the PR interval on the ECG, the A wave sequence on the CVP waveform represents atrial contraction.

The X descent on the CVP waveform represents atrial relaxation and declining pressure after systole, when the atrium expels blood into the ventricle.

As the cardiac cycle progresses, the tricuspid valve closes, producing a small backward bulge known as the C wave.

The atrium filling with venous blood during diastole produces another rise in pressure and a V wave, which corresponds to the T wave of the ECG.

After atrial filling, the tricuspid valve opens. Most of the blood in the right atrium passively empties into the right ventricle, causing atrial pressure to fall. On the CVP waveform, this decline appears as the Y descent.

The A and V waves are almost the same height, indicating that atrial systole and atrial diastole produce about the same amount of pressure. Consequently, right atrial pressures are recorded as mean values because they're almost the same.

What causes rising waves?

Conditions that cause increased resistance to ventricular filling, such as heart failure or tricuspid stenosis, generate elevated A waves.

Elevated V waves result from regurgitant flow—for example, from tricuspid insufficiency or from inadequate closure of the tricuspid valve due to heart failure. Although the V wave may be elevated in tricuspid insufficiency, its height doesn't correspond to the amount of regurgitant flow.

Elevations in the A and V waves may result from cardiac tamponade, constrictive pericardial disease, or heart failure. Increased resistance to ventricular filling causes the elevated A wave; functional regurgitation causes the elevated V wave.

What causes descending waves?

Cardiac tamponade causes a smaller Y descent than an X descent. This results partly from an increase in heart rate and the right atrium's inability to empty efficiently because of the blood backflow that occurs with tamponade.

If the patient has a disorder causing constrictive pericardial disease, the Y descent exceeds the X descent. In such cases, ventricular filling occurs rapidly, producing the exaggerated Y deflection.

MONITORING C.V.P. WITH A WATER MANOMETER

Using a water manometer to monitor central venous pressure (CVP) requires setting up the equipment and connecting it to the patient's central venous catheter before recording pressure measurements.

Typically, the patient already has the catheter in place—to administer I.V. therapy, for example—and the I.V. line that you'll use to measure CVP will connect to it. The manometer is plastic and disposable. A three- or four-way stopcock connects the manometer to the I.V. line leading to the catheter. The manometer's plastic column has graduated markings, allowing pressure values to be measured in centimeters of water (cm H_2O).

Setting up the manometer

Assemble the following equipment: a CVP water manometer with stopcock, the prescribed I.V. solution, an I.V. administration set, gloves, tape, a marking pen, and a carpenter's level or ruler. Additionally, you will need an I.V. pole. If you expect to draw blood samples for analysis, you'll need an extra stopcock. Take the equipment to the patient's bedside.

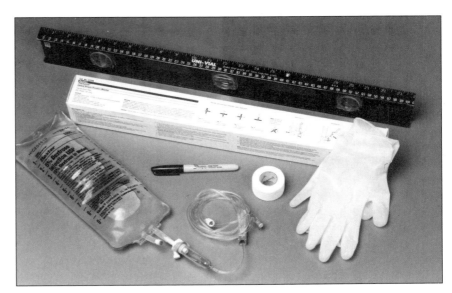

Explain the procedure to the patient, and answer his questions to help allay his fears. After washing your hands, remove the manometer from its package.

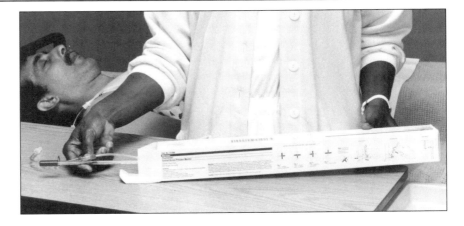

Connect the I.V. administration set to the prescribed I.V. solution. Check all connections to make sure that they're tight. This helps prevent contamination and disconnections.

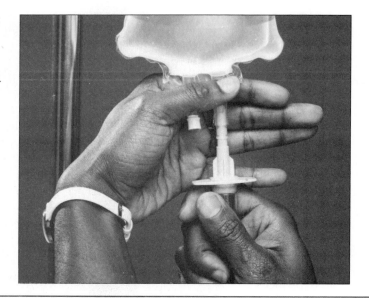

Prime the tubing with the I.V. solution just as you would any I.V. administration set. Make sure that no air remains in the tubing before you attach it to the patient's central venous catheter.

▶ *Clinical tip:* Once you finish assembling the monitoring equipment, you can minimize the potential for contamination by maintaining the connections between the I.V. tubing and the manometer and between the manometer and the patient's central venous catheter.

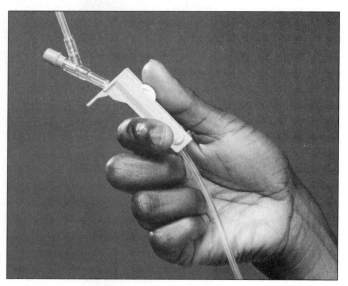

Attach the I.V. tubing to one side of the manometer stopcock. Prime the manometer by turning the stopcock so that it's closed to the patient and open to the manometer.

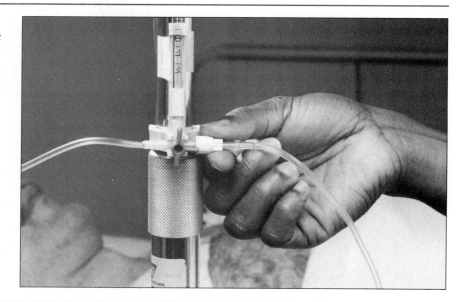

Open the roller clamp, and slowly let the manometer column fill to about the 20-cm mark. Don't over-fill the manometer. Although the markings on the manometer differ according to the manufacturer, they typically range from −2 cm to 38 cm. To avoid problems, read the directions that come with the manometer before assembling the equipment and taking readings.

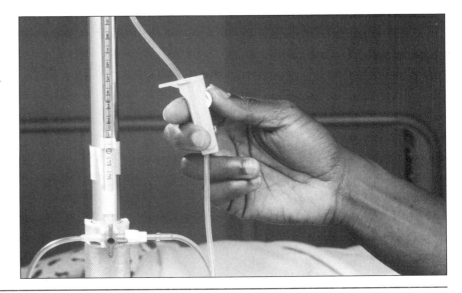

Connecting the manometer to the catheter

Have the patient lie flat in bed or in a slight Trendelenburg position. This engorges the blood vessels and helps counteract the negative intrathoracic pressure caused by connecting (or reconnecting) the manometer to the central venous catheter.

▶ *Clinical tip:* Have the patient perform Valsalva's maneu-ver while you connect the manom-eter and the central venous cathe-ter. This may help to prevent an air embolism from developing when the catheter lumen is ex-posed briefly to atmospheric air.

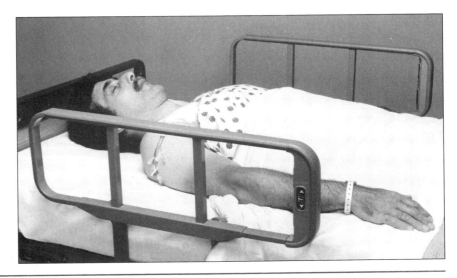

Put on gloves. Then clamp the central venous catheter and uncap the lumen. If you expect to draw blood samples, add another stop-cock to the hub of the central ve-nous catheter (as shown). This will also help you when attaching the central venous catheter to the manometer. Afterward, flush all the ports with I.V. solution and place a nonvented cap on the un-used vertical port.

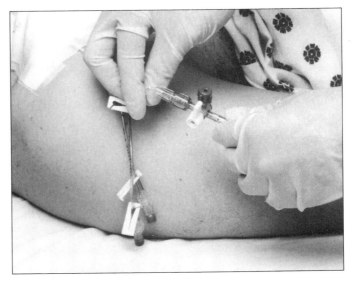

If you attached an additional stopcock to the hub, close it to the patient. Then remove the cap on the other end of the stopcock, and attach the manometer tubing to that end.

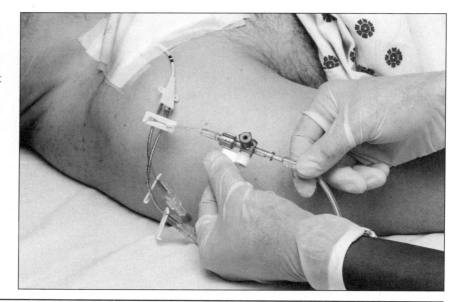

Alternatively, if you're not using an additional stopcock, quickly attach the manometer's fluid-filled connecting tubing to the hub of the central venous catheter. Be careful to maintain the sterility of the hub and tubing. Next, unclamp the central venous catheter.

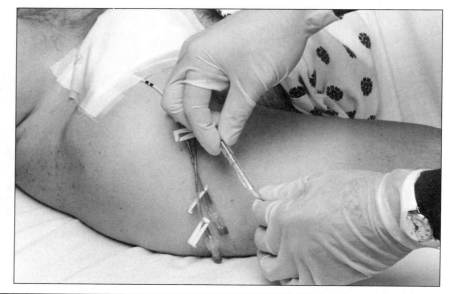

After you connect the manometer tubing to the catheter hub or the additional stopcock, turn the stopcock to the open position—that is, closed to the manometer and open to the patient. This creates a direct line from the I.V. set to the patient. Open the I.V. roller clamp (as shown) to ensure adequate fluid flow, and adjust the flow rate. Now you're ready to take pressure readings. Remove your gloves and wash your hands.

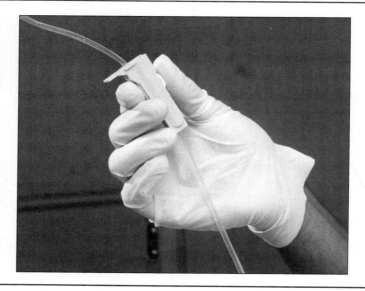

Measuring CVP

Have the patient lie flat in bed without a pillow. If he can't tolerate this position, raise the head of the bed slightly—but no higher than 30 degrees. If a completely different position needs to be used, note this on the chart. Be sure to take all subsequent pressure readings with the patient in the same position.

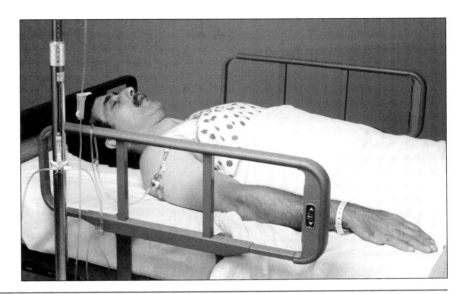

Locate the patient's phlebostatic axis (the level of the right atrium) by mentally bisecting the fourth intercostal space at the midpoint of the anteroposterior chest wall. (Or use the midaxillary line, but be aware that pressure readings may be less accurate.) Put a piece of tape on the patient's side, and use a marking pen to pinpoint the phlebostatic axis.

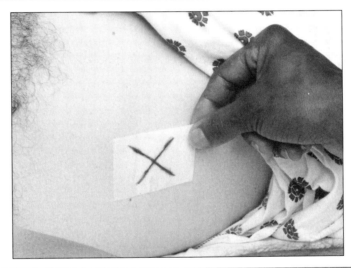

Next, attach the manometer to an I.V. pole at the bedside, or place the manometer next to the patient. Align the zero mark on the manometer with the phlebostatic axis. Use a device such as a carpenter's level to ensure a level alignment.

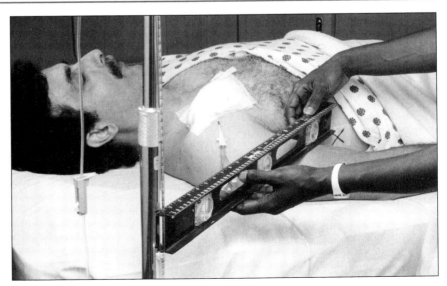

To check the central venous catheter for patency, open the roller clamp on the I.V. tubing and watch for the I.V. solution to flow freely.

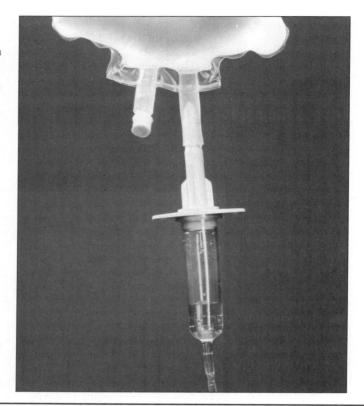

If you doubt the catheter's patency, check for obvious kinking. If you don't see any kinking, put on gloves, attach a syringe to the catheter or stopcock, and try to aspirate blood according to hospital policy. If blood enters the syringe, reinfuse the blood and infuse the I.V. solution again. If you can't aspirate blood, suspect a blockage and notify the doctor. Don't irrigate the catheter. If the patient has a blood clot, irrigation could dislodge it.

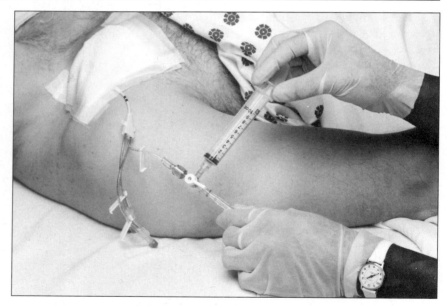

Turn the stopcock so that the I.V. solution runs into the manometer. Fill the manometer with I.V. solution by opening the roller clamp and filling the column with 10 to 20 ml of fluid above the normal range.

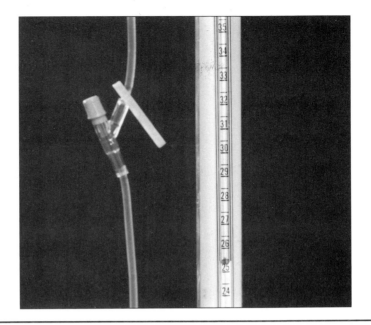

Next, close the stopcock to the I.V. solution and open it to the patient.

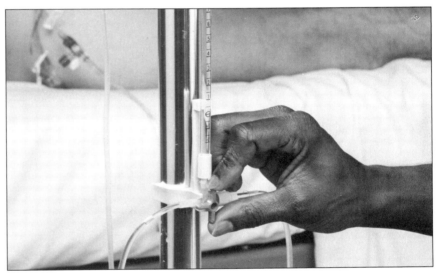

As the patient breathes, observe the fluid level in the manometer column. On inspiration, the level should fall; on expiration, the level should rise slightly. Note the point at which the falling fluid level comes to rest and fluctuates only slightly with respirations. This is end-expiration in the respiratory cycle.

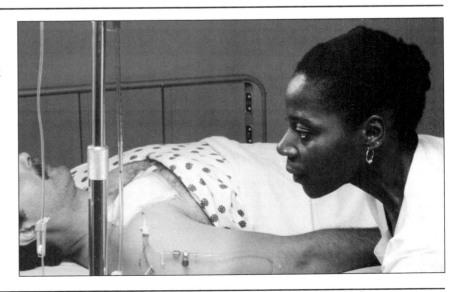

Once you recognize end-expiration, take a CVP reading. The correct value is at the bottom of the meniscus (the low point in the water curve in the manometer).

▶ *Clinical tip:* If small air bubbles appear trapped in the manometer, tap the manometer column lightly to dislodge them. After you remove all of the air bubbles, read the CVP value.

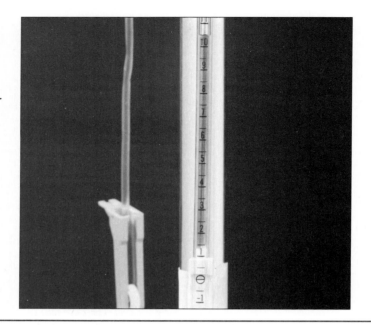

After obtaining the reading, turn the stopcock so that the I.V. solution can be infused. Reset the I.V. flow rate at the appropriate infusion rate, and reposition the patient for comfort. Document the patient's response to the procedure and the values obtained.

▶ *Clinical tip:* When you monitor CVP continuously, you'll leave the I.V. solution stopcock open. When you review the patient's readings, keep in mind that the pressure of the I.V. solution infusing will raise the CVP values slightly (although the patient's CVP won't actually be increased). If you infuse the I.V. solution at a constant rate, the pressure values will still reflect changes in the patient's condition.

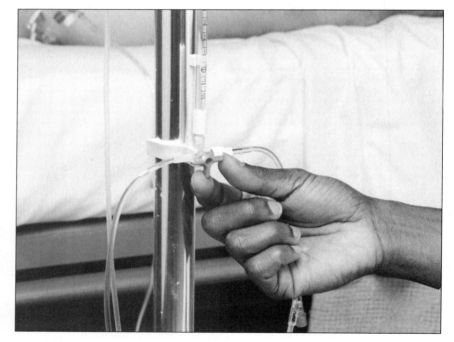

LEARNING ABOUT CARDIAC OUTPUT MONITORING

Measuring cardiac output—the volume of blood ejected from the heart over 1 minute—helps evaluate cardiac function. Normally, cardiac output ranges from 4 to 8 liters/minute. Values below this range result from:
• decreased myocardial contractility caused by myocardial infarction, drug effects, acidosis, or hypoxia
• decreased left ventricular filling pressure resulting from hypovolemia
• increased systemic vascular resistance related to arteriosclerosis or hypertension
• decreased ventricular flow related to valvular heart disease.

High cardiac output can occur with some arteriovenous shunts and from decreased vascular resistance (as in septic shock). In some cases, an unusually high cardiac output can be normal (for example, in well-conditioned athletes).

Cardiac output values along with mean arterial pressure, right atrial pressure, mean pulmonary artery pressure, and pulmonary artery wedge pressure can also provide further information about cardiovascular function—for example, stroke volume and vascular resistance.

REVIEWING MEASURING METHODS

Indirect methods of measuring cardiac output include the Fick method, the indicator-dilution method, and the thermodilution method. The Fick and indicator-dilution methods are performed mostly in cardiac catheterization laboratories or in research projects.

Fick method
Effective for detecting low cardiac output, the Fick method calculates cardiac output (CO) by measuring oxygen levels in the blood before and after the blood passes through the lungs and, using a spirometer, by measuring oxygen consumption—the amount of air entering the lungs each minute, as follows:

$$\text{CO (liter/min)} = \frac{\text{oxygen consumption (cc/min)}}{\text{arterial oxygen content (ml/min)} - \text{venous oxygen content (ml/min)}}$$

A drawback to this procedure is that the patient must be in a steady physiologic state. Most patients requiring cardiac output determinations are critically ill, which is frequently defined as an "unsteady state." This technique also requires simultaneous expired air and blood samples, controlled inspired oxygen content values, and arterial blood samples.

Indicator-dilution method
This method uses a computer to evaluate cardiac output. Computations involve measuring the volume and concentration of an injected dye indicator as it passes from the pulmonary artery to the brachial artery over a certain time. The results are plotted as a time and dilution-concentration curve.

The drawback of this technique is that it requires complex equipment skills to obtain accurate results and, therefore, is not a clinically practical method.

Thermodilution method
Used at bedside, the thermodilution method applies indicator-dilution principles, using temperature changes in the pulmonary artery blood as the indicator. The procedure requires the addition of a thermistor (a temperature sensor) onto the pulmonary artery catheter. Thermodilution monitoring is relatively easy, rapid (values can be computed approximately every minute), and clean (no blood sampling is required).

CALCULATING THE CARDIAC INDEX

Because it takes into account the patient's size, the cardiac index is a more accurate indicator of cardiac output. To calculate the cardiac index, divide the cardiac output value by the patient's body surface area (BSA). Normally, the cardiac index ranges from 2.5 to 4 liters/minute/m² (of BSA).

You can obtain the patient's BSA by plotting his height and weight on the Du Bois BSA nomogram. This chart consists of three columns. Mark the patient's height on the scale in column one and his weight in column three. Then draw a line linking these two points. The point at which your line intercepts column two indicates the patient's estimated BSA.

Jan Headley, RN, BS, and *Loraine Hopkins Pepe, RN, MSN, CCRN, CS,* contributed to this section. Ms. Headley is a senior education consultant for Baxter Healthcare Corp., Edwards Critical-Care Division, Irvine, Calif. Ms. Pepe is a staff nurse in the medical-surgical intensive care unit at Chestnut Hill Hospital, Philadelphia. The publisher thanks the following organizations for their help: *Baxter Healthcare Corp., Edwards Critical-Care Division,* Irvine, Calif.; *Doylestown (Pa.) Hospital; Hewlett-Packard Co.,* Waltham, Mass.; and *Hill-Rom,* Batesville, Ind.

Another method used to calculate BSA is the Boyd method. This method uses a formula to calculate BSA for children and for adults with a large body mass. The DuBois and Boyd methods generally have similar results except when BSA is very large. Although these two methods are popular, several other methods for calculating BSA exist. Many bedside computers can also calculate the patient's BSA when you enter the patient's height and weight. Check your hospital's policy to determine which method to use.

UNDERSTANDING THERMODILUTION MONITORING

In thermodilution monitoring, a balloon-tipped, flow-directed catheter is inserted into a large vein, advanced to the right side of the heart, and positioned in the pulmonary artery. You'll inject a specific amount of solution called an injectate (at a specific temperature) into the proximal port of the pulmonary artery catheter. (Depending on your equipment, you can also use the right atrium—or the lumen marked RA.)

As the injectate mixes with the surrounding blood and flows into the pulmonary artery, a thermistor embedded in the catheter senses the temperature change and a bedside computer plots the change. This plotting, known as a time-temperature (thermodilution) curve, contains the information needed to calculate the cardiac output. Once the computer processes the data, results appear on the monitor. Some monitors display the actual thermodilution curve.

Several factors must be considered during thermodilution monitoring: the injectate type and temperature, the correct selection of a computation constant, and the type of delivery system.

Injectate: Type and temperature

Dextrose 5% in water (D_5W) is the recommended I.V. solution because the computation constant is based in part on this solution's specific gravity and temperature response. Using 0.9% sodium chloride solution instead produces a 2% decrease in the cardiac output value.

The injectate may be room temperature or iced. Because researchers show conflicting results when comparing room-temperature and iced injectates and their impact on cardiac output readings, follow your hospital's policy when preparing the injectate for your patient.

Computation constant

The computation constant accounts for the gain of heat from the catheter tubing as injectate travels through the catheter into the blood. Its selection is based on such variables as the volume and temperature of the injectate as well as the size and type of catheter you plan to use. Usually the catheter manufacturer supplies the computation constant values (sometimes in chart form). Verify this number any time you change one of the variables. Most bedside computers require you to alter the computation constant manually, although some have sensing capabilities that can detect changes in the variables.

Keep in mind that an inaccurate computation constant can produce an error of up to 100% in the cardiac output value. Also, if you change the injectate volume from 5 to 10 ml without changing the computation constant, the resulting cardiac output value may differ significantly from the true value.

Delivery systems

Besides having a choice of injectates and temperatures when using the thermodilution method, you'll also have a choice of delivery systems: closed and open. Each system works with room-temperature or iced injectate.

PERFORMING CLOSED THERMODILUTION MONITORING

If you select the closed system, you'll use one syringe to feed injectate into the bloodstream via the catheter in a closed-loop system. The closed system reduces the risk of contamination inherent in the open system by eliminating the need for multiple entry into a sterile system.

You'll need a bolus injectate system (such as the Baxter CO-Set shown here, which includes a cooling container, coiled tubing, and an insulated 10-ml syringe), injectate (a 500-ml bag of D_5W or 0.9% sodium chloride solution), a thermistor, connecting cables, and a stopcock. If you're using iced injectate, obtain the ice and water.

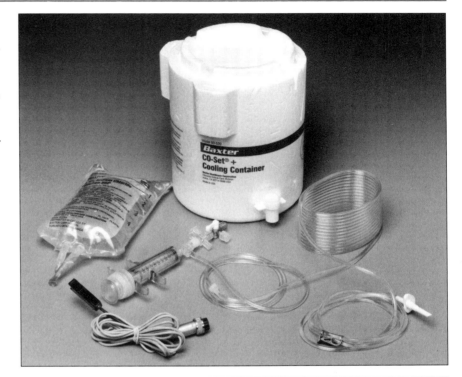

You'll also need a cardiac output computer or a module for the bedside monitor.

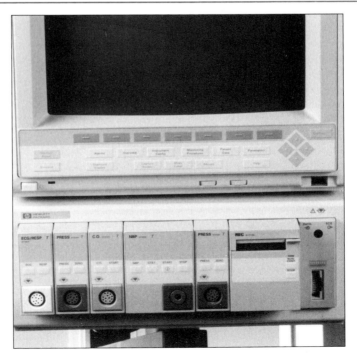

Take the equipment to the patient's bedside. Explain the procedure and wash your hands. Plug the connecting cable into the cardiac output module.

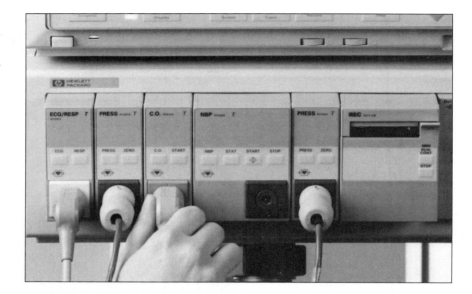

Then plug the catheter connector into the thermistor connector of the pulmonary artery (PA) catheter.

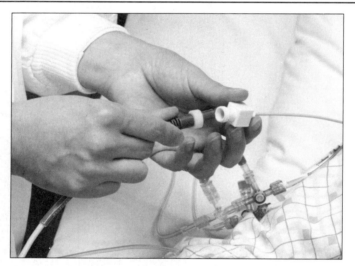

Press the module's CARDIAC OUTPUT key. A computation constant number will appear on the display screen (as shown). Consult the manufacturer's instructions to make sure that this number is appropriate for the injectate, its temperature range, and the type of catheter you're using.

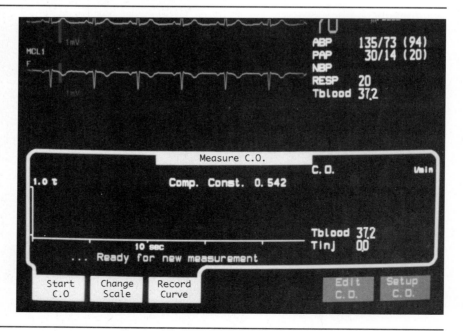

Check to see that two stopcocks are in place on the catheter's proximal lumen. If they're not, attach two now. Both stopcocks should be turned off to the capped end (as shown).

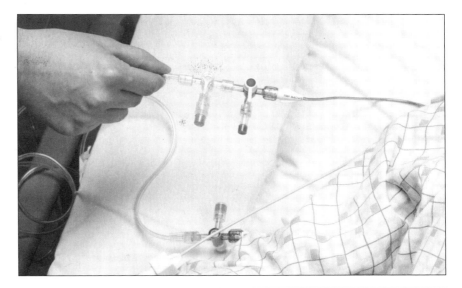

Next, observe the pulmonary artery pressure (PAP) waveform on the monitor to verify that the PA catheter is properly positioned with the balloon tip deflated. An improperly positioned catheter may produce inaccurate cardiac output values.

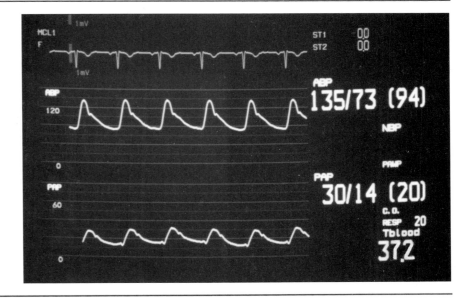

Though some hospital policies require the patient to lie flat, your hospital may permit the patient to lie supine with his head slightly elevated (but no more than 30 degrees). Document the patient's exact position on his chart so that he lies in the same position for future cardiac output measurements.

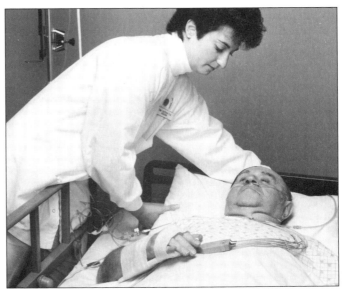

Attach the I.V. solution bag to the injectate delivery system. To prime the system, unclamp the snap clamp on the I.V. tubing and allow the solution to flow through the tubing. Slowly pull the syringe plunger out and then push it in (as shown) to remove any air. Repeat this procedure five to six times to ensure that the system is free of air. Then place the cooling container on the I.V. pole.

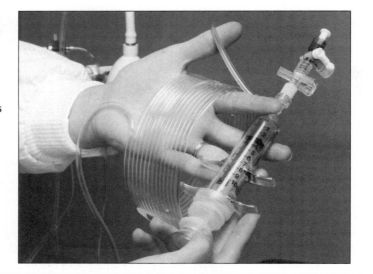

Close the clamp once you've primed the tubing. Place the coiled portion of the tubing into the cooling container (as shown). If you're cooling the injectate, make sure that the iced solution surrounds the coil. If you're using room-temperature injectate, don't place the coiled tubing in the cooling container.

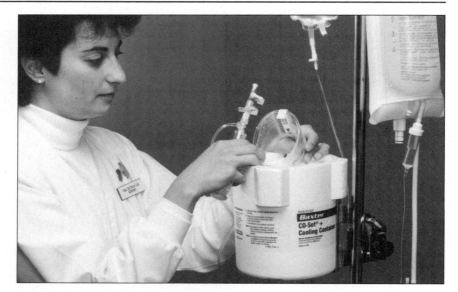

Next, put on gloves and attach the system to the stopcock closest to the catheter's proximal lumen.

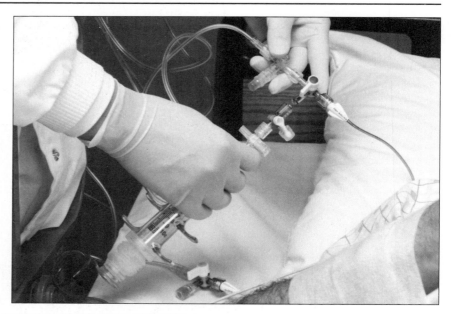

Attach the in-line temperature probe to the hub on the closed system set.

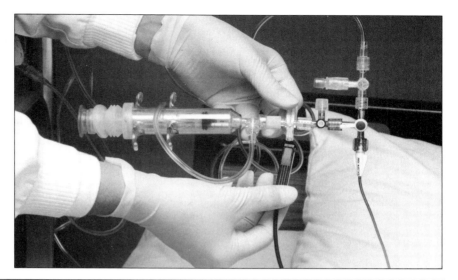

Make sure that the stopcock closest to the catheter's proximal lumen is closed (as shown).

Depending on your hospital's policy, the proximal lumen may be reserved for cardiac output measurements. However, it may need a continuous-drip infusion line if medications will be administered to the patient intermittently through it. If this is the case, attach a prepared continuous-drip infusion line to the second stopcock and close this stopcock to the pressure side of the proximal lumen (to suspend any concurrent pressure waveform measurements).

▶ *Clinical tip:* If the proximal lumen isn't reserved for cardiac output measurement, avoid using this site to infuse vasoactive agents or other medications that can't be discontinued temporarily.

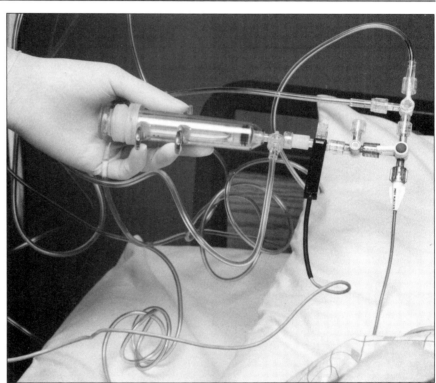

Open the snap clamp on the I.V. solution tubing.

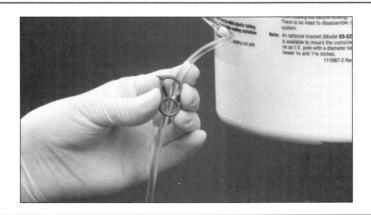

Carefully withdraw exactly 10 ml of injectate into the insulated syringe attached to the proximal lumen. Be aware that an error in the injectate volume can produce an error in the cardiac output value. (For example, injecting 11 ml instead of 10 ml can produce a 10% error.)

▶ *Clinical tip:* If you're using an uninsulated syringe barrel, avoid excessive handling, which may warm a room-temperature injectate 1° C (1.8° F) in 28 seconds and an iced injectate 1° C in 13 seconds. A 1° C change in the delivered injectate temperature can produce an error of 2.8% or more in the cardiac output value.

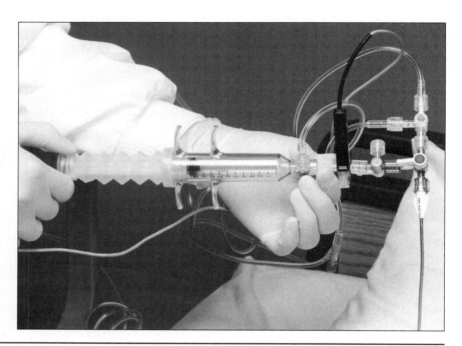

Press the START key on the monitor module. When the monitor indicates that it's ready, observe the patient's breathing (as shown) and instill the injectate rapidly and smoothly during the end-expiratory phase of the respiratory cycle. The injection should take no more than 4 seconds to complete. If your monitor displays the thermodilution curve, look for a smooth and sharp rise in the curve.

Be sure to instill the injectate during the end-expiratory phase each time you perform the procedure to ensure reliable and consistent results.

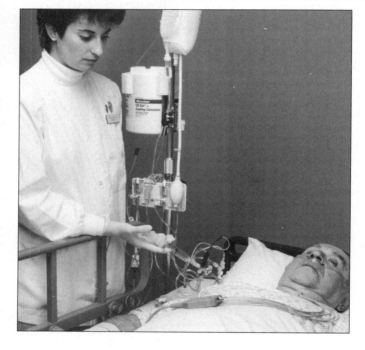

Check the injectate's temperature on the monitor during or immediately after injection. Iced injectate should measure between 6° and 12° C (42.8° and 53.6° F). Room-temperature injectate should measure between 18° and 25° C (64.4° and 77° F), or at least 10° C (18° F) below the patient's blood temperature.

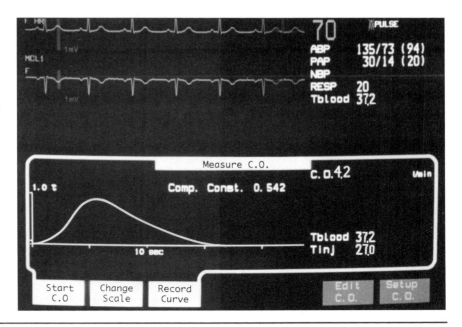

Repeat the injection procedure at least three times—more if necessary—to obtain a mean cardiac output value. Discard any reading that isn't within 10% of the other readings.

When you finish the procedure, close the snap clamp on the injectate solution line.

▶ ***Clinical tip:*** Be sure to close the snap clamp. If you forget to do so and then hang the injectate bag on an I.V. pole, gravity will force the solution into the syringe; this will result in inconsistent injectate temperatures, requiring you to repeat the procedure from the beginning.

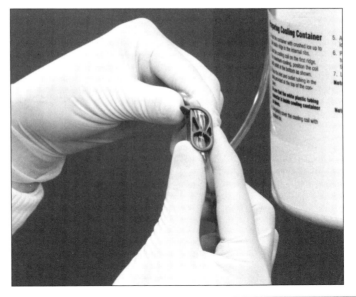

Turn the stopcock to the open position so that the pressure flush from the I.V. solution will keep the line patent. If the lumen you were using to measure cardiac output was also being used to monitor right atrial pressure (RAP), observe the monitor for the return of an RAP waveform. Then reposition the patient if necessary to make him more comfortable.

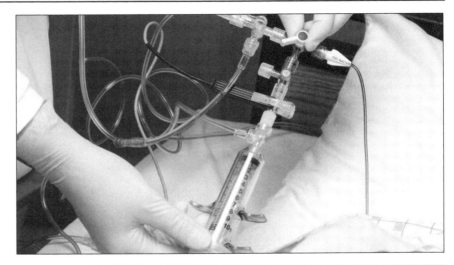

Average the readings to obtain the mean cardiac output value. Typically, an individual reading within 10% of the other readings is considered acceptable and representative of the patient's condition.

If you repeatedly obtain individual values that deviate by more than 10% from the others, you may have to reassess the patient's condition, double-check your technique, and repeat the procedure.

Record the mean cardiac output value on the patient's chart. Be sure to describe how the patient tolerated the procedure.

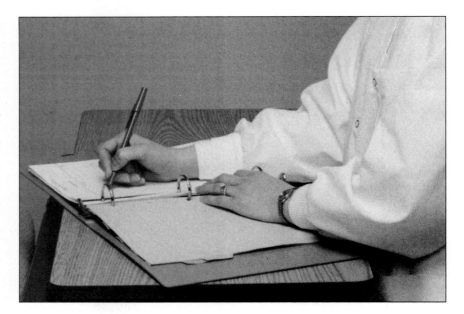

PERFORMING OPEN THERMODILUTION MONITORING

If you select the open system of thermodilution monitoring, you'll use several prefilled syringes, attaching a new syringe to the catheter lumen each time you instill injectate.

You'll need an injectate temperature sensor or cable, the injectate (a 250-ml or 500-ml bag of D₅W or 0.9% sodium chloride solution), a stopcock, five 10-ml syringes with 1″ or 1½″ 20G needles, an insulated container, a plastic bag, and an alcohol pad. If you're using iced injectate, obtain the ice and water.

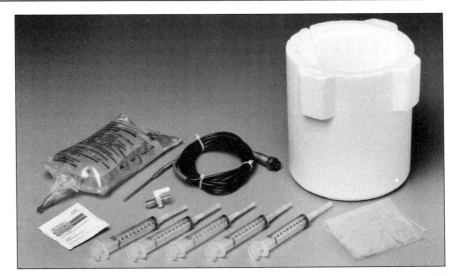

You'll also need a cardiac output computer or a module for the bedside monitor.

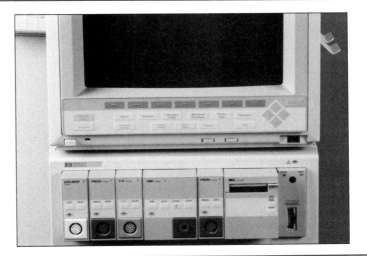

Take the necessary equipment to the patient's bedside. Explain the procedure and wash your hands. Plug the connecting cable into the cardiac output module. Then plug the catheter connector into the thermistor connector of the PA catheter (as shown).

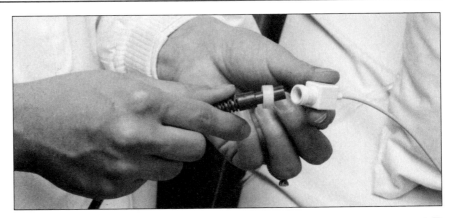

Press the module's CARDIAC OUTPUT key. A computation constant number will appear on the display screen. Verify that the computation constant is correct for the catheter type and for the volume and temperature of the injectate you'll be using. Reset the computation constant if necessary.

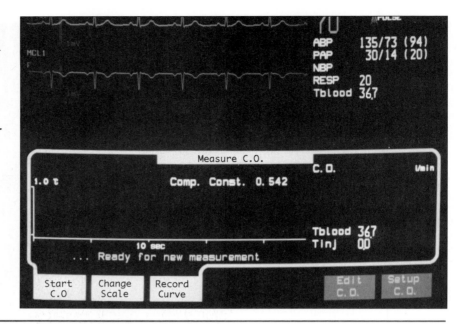

Don gloves. If a stopcock isn't already in place on the catheter's proximal lumen, quickly attach one now. Don't allow air to enter the catheter.

▶ *Clinical tip:* Be sure to avoid infusing medications (especially vasoactive drugs) through the RA lumen before instilling the injectate. Doing so could alter the cardiac output reading.

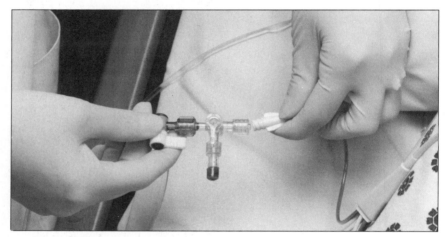

Observe the pulmonary artery pressure (PAP) waveform on the monitor to verify that the catheter is correctly positioned and that the balloon tip is deflated. An improperly positioned catheter may produce inaccurate cardiac output values.

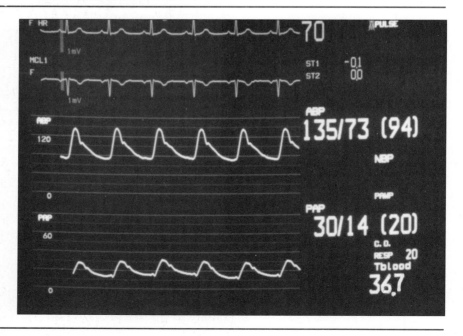

Place the patient in a supine position. Depending on your hospital's policy, you may elevate the head of the bed up to 30 degrees for patient comfort. Record the patient's exact position on her chart to serve as a reference for future cardiac output measurements.

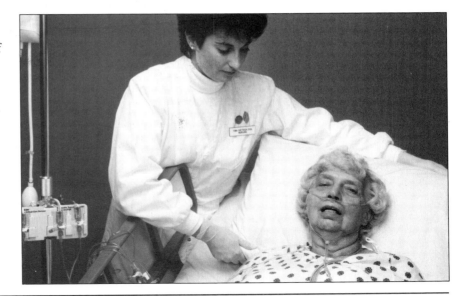

If you're using iced injectate, fill an insulated container with ice and water.

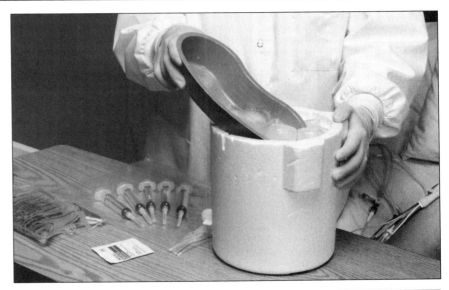

Wipe the injection port of the I.V. bag with an alcohol pad. Then draw exactly 10 ml of injectate from the I.V. bag into each of the five 10-ml syringes.

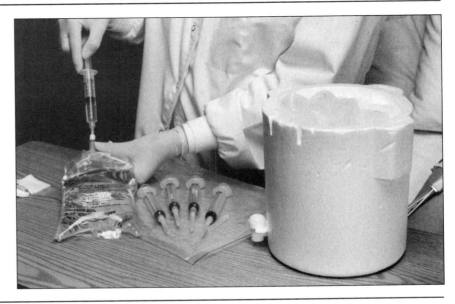

Remove the plunger from one of the syringes. Place the injectate temperature sensor inside the syringe as you put the syringe in the ice solution.

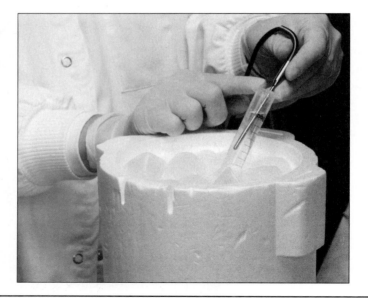

Put the remaining four syringes in the plastic bag.

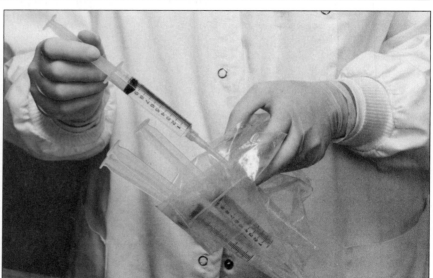

Then place the bag of syringes in the ice solution. The bag will protect the injectate from possible contamination from the ice. During the procedure, the syringe with the sensor will monitor the temperature of the injectate in all the syringes. After the procedure, you'll discard this syringe.

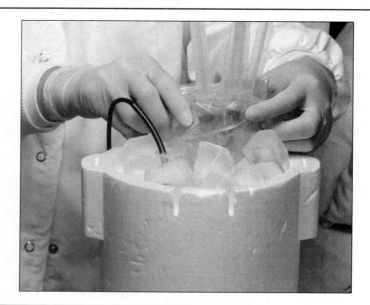

Allow the syringes to chill. Then observe the monitor to ensure that the injectate temperature remains steady at 6° to 12° C (42.8° to 53.6° F).

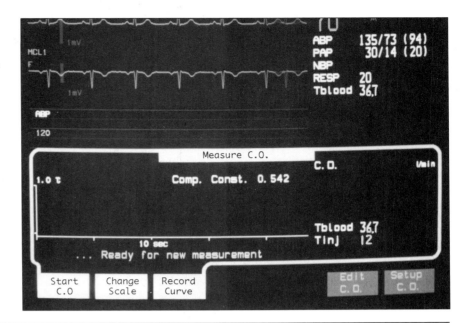

If you're using room-temperature injectate, make sure that the injectate temperature remains between 18° and 25° C (64.4° and 77° F) or at least 10° C (18° F) below blood temperature. Remove the plunger from one of the filled syringes and place the temperature sensor inside. (This syringe will be discarded after the procedure.) Observe the temperature on the monitor.

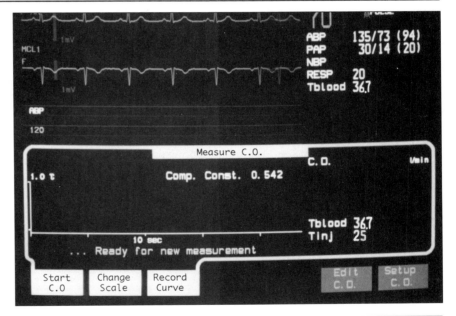

Attach one of the prefilled syringes to the stopcock on the proximal lumen. Turn the stopcock so that it's closed to the I.V. infusion or pressure flush and open to the catheter.

▶ *Clinical tip:* Avoid prolonged handling of the syringe because this may warm the injectate and alter the cardiac output values.

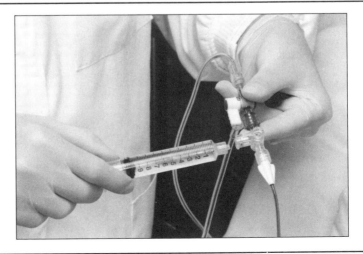

Press the module's START key. When the monitor indicates that it's ready, rapidly and smoothly instill the injectate within 4 seconds during the end-expiratory phase of the respiratory cycle.

▶ *Clinical tip:* Because blood flow varies during the respiratory cycle, instill the injectate during the same phase of the cycle each time you perform the procedure to ensure consistent and accurate results.

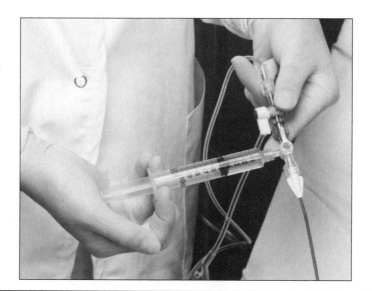

If your monitor displays a thermo-dilution curve, watch for a smooth and sharp rise initiating the curve. Continue to observe the curve as you repeat the injection procedure at least three times. Discard any reading that isn't within 10% of the other readings.

You'll need at least three readings to obtain a reliable mean value—four or more if you have to discard a reading outside the acceptable 10% range. If you repeatedly obtain individual values that vary by more than 10%, reassess the patient's condition, double-check your technique, and repeat the procedure.

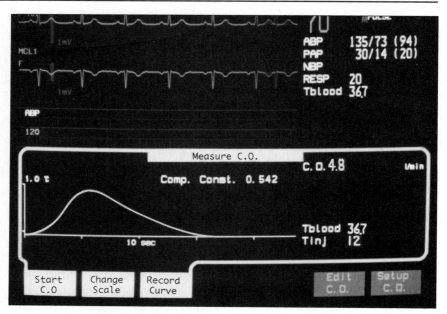

When the procedure is complete, turn the stopcock so that it's open to the I.V. infusion or pressure flush. If the lumen you were using was also being used to monitor the right atrium, observe the monitor for the return of a right atrial pressure waveform. Then place the patient in a comfortable position.

Average the readings to obtain a mean cardiac output value. Document this value and the patient's tolerance of the procedure.

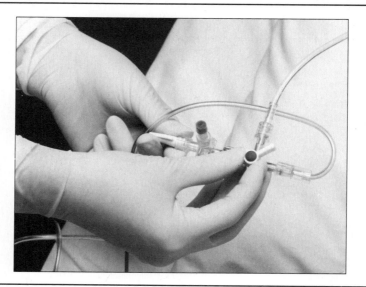

Measuring cardiac functions

To measure various aspects of cardiac function, combine cardiac output values with other key values obtainable when the patient has a pulmonary artery line and a separate arterial line. These values include mean arterial pressure, right atrial pressure, mean pulmonary artery pressure, and pulmonary artery wedge pressure. Then calculate stroke volume, stroke volume index, systemic vascular resistance, or pulmonary vascular resistance using the formulas below. For continuity, the same values for cardiac output (CO), heart rate (HR), and stroke volume (SV) will be used throughout the equations.

Keep in mind that some monitoring systems compute these values automatically.

Stroke volume

To determine SV—the volume of blood pumped by the ventricle in one contraction—multiply the CO by 1,000 and divide by the HR. Normal SV ranges between 60 and 100 ml/beat. Use this equation:

$$SV = \frac{CO \times 1,000}{HR}$$

Example: Here the patient's CO is 5.5 liters/minute and his HR is 80 beats/minute.

$$SV = \frac{5.5 \times 1,000}{80} = \frac{5,500}{80} = 68.75 \text{ ml/beat}$$

Stroke volume index

To assess whether the patient's SV is adequate for his body size, compute the stroke volume index (SVI). Do this either by dividing the SV by the patient's body surface area (BSA) or by dividing his cardiac index (CI) by his HR. Normally, the SVI ranges between 33 and 47 ml/beat/m² of BSA. Use either of these equations:

$$SVI = \frac{SV}{BSA} \text{ or } \frac{CI}{HR}$$

Example: As we determined in the example above, the patient's SV is 68.75 ml/beat. His BSA is 1.64 m² and his CI (calculated by dividing his CO by his BSA) is 3.35 liters/min/m².

$$SVI = \frac{SV}{BSA} = \frac{68.75}{1.64} = 42 \text{ ml/beat/m}^2$$

or

$$SVI = \frac{CI}{HR} = \frac{3.35}{80} = 0.042 \text{ liters/beat/m}^2$$

Systemic vascular resistance

To assess systemic vascular resistance (SVR)—the degree of left ventricular resistance known as afterload—deduct right atrial pressure (RAP) from mean arterial pressure (MAP). Then multiply by a rounded conversion factor of 80 to commute the value into units of force (dynes/sec/cm⁻⁵). Divide this value by the CO value.

Many hospitals consider a range of 800 to 1,200 dynes/sec/cm⁻⁵ to be a normal SVR value; however, the American Association of Critical-Care Nurses (AACN) accepts 900 to 1,400 dynes/sec/cm⁻⁵ as a normal range. To do your own calculations, use this equation:

$$SVR = \frac{(MAP - RAP) \times 80}{CO}$$

Example: Here the patient's MAP is 93 and his RAP is 6; CO remains 5.5. Note that 80 is the conversion factor.

$$SVR = \frac{(93 - 6) \times 80}{5.5} = \frac{6,960}{5.5} = 1,265 \text{ dynes/sec/cm}^{-5}$$

Pulmonary vascular resistance

To measure pulmonary vascular resistance (PVR)—or right ventricular afterload—deduct pulmonary artery wedge pressure (PAWP) from mean pulmonary artery pressure (MPAP). To commute the value into units of force (dynes/sec/cm⁻⁵), multiply the result by a rounded conversion factor of 80. Then divide the product by the CO value.

According to the AACN, the normal range for PVR is 155 to 255 dynes/sec/cm⁻⁵. To calculate your patient's PVR, use this equation:

$$PVR = \frac{(MPAP - PAWP) \times 80}{CO}$$

Example: Here the patient's MPAP is 20 and his PAWP is 5; his CO remains 5.5. Again the conversion factor is 80.

$$PVR = \frac{(20 - 5) \times 80}{5.5} = \frac{1,200}{5.5} = 218 \text{ dynes/sec/cm}^{-5}$$

INSIGHTS AND INTERPRETATIONS

Analyzing thermodilution curves

The thermodilution curve provides valuable information about cardiac output, injection technique, and equipment problems. When studying the curve, keep in mind that the area under the curve is inversely proportional to cardiac output: The smaller the area under the curve, the higher the cardiac output; the larger the area under the curve, the lower the cardiac output.

Besides providing a record of cardiac output, the curve may indicate problems related to technique, such as erratic or slow injectate instillations, or other problems, such as respiratory variations or electrical interference. The curves below correspond to those typically seen in clinical practice.

Normal thermodilution curve

With an accurate monitoring system and a patient who has adequate cardiac output, the thermodilution curve begins with a smooth, rapid upstroke and is followed by a smooth, gradual downslope. The curve shown below indicates that the injectate instillation time was within the recommended 4 seconds and that the temperature curve returned to baseline blood temperature.

The height of the curve will vary, depending on whether you use a room-temperature or an iced injectate. Room-temperature injectate produces an upstroke of lower amplitude.

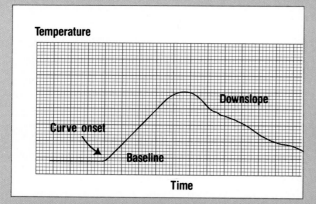

Low-cardiac-output curve

A thermodilution curve representing low cardiac output shows a rapid, smooth upstroke (from proper injection technique). But because the heart is ejecting blood less efficiently from the ventricles, the injectate warms slowly and takes longer to be ejected from the ventricle. Consequently, the curve takes longer to return to baseline. This slow return produces a larger area under the curve, corresponding to low cardiac output.

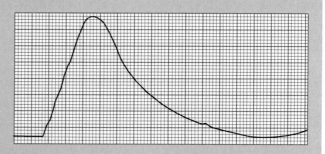

High-cardiac-output curve

Again, the curve has a rapid, smooth upstroke from proper injection technique. But because the ventricles are ejecting blood too forcefully, the injectate moves through the heart quickly and the curve returns to baseline more rapidly. The smaller area under the curve suggests higher cardiac output.

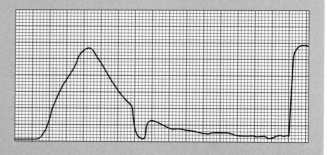

Analyzing thermodilution curves *(continued)*

Curve reflecting poor technique

This curve results from an uneven and too slow (taking more than 4 seconds) administration of injectate. The uneven and slower-than-normal upstroke and the larger area under the curve erroneously indicate low cardiac output. A kinked catheter, unsteady hands during the injection, or improper placement of the injectate lumen in the introducer sheath may also cause this type of curve.

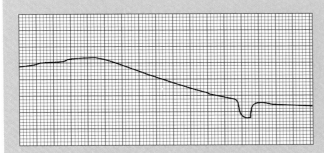

Curve associated with respiratory variations

To obtain a reliable cardiac output measurement, you need a steady baseline pulmonary artery blood temperature. If the patient has rapid or labored respirations, or if he's receiving mechanical ventilation, the thermodilution curve may reflect inaccurate cardiac output values. The curve below from a patient receiving mechanical ventilation reflects fluctuating pulmonary artery blood temperatures. The thermistor interprets the unsteady temperature as a return to baseline. The result is a curve erroneously showing high cardiac output (small area under the curve).

Note: In some cases, the equipment senses no return to baseline at all and produces a sinelike curve recorded by the computer as 0.00.

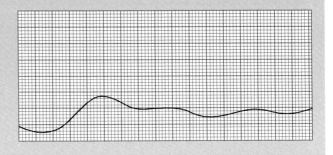

Correcting problems of cardiac output monitoring

PROBLEM	CAUSES	INTERVENTIONS
Cardiac output values lower than expected	Injectate volume greater than indicated for computation constant	• Be sure to instill only the injectate volume that's appropriate for the computation constant.
	Erroneous computation constant (set too low)	• Before injection, verify that the computation constant setting and the injectate volume are compatible. • To avoid repeating the injection procedure, correct the cardiac output (CO) value and the computation constant (CC) setting. To do so, use this formula: CO wrong × CC right ÷ CC wrong = CO right. Then reset the monitor for the next serial injection, using the correct computation constant.
	Injectate lumen exits in right ventricle	• Confirm proper placement of the injectate lumen by observing the monitor for right atrial waveforms.
Cardiac output values higher than expected	Injectate volume smaller than indicated for computation constant	• Before injection, verify that the injectate volume is correct for the determined computation constant. • Look for and expel air bubbles from the injectate syringe.
	Erroneous computation constant (set too high)	• Before injection, verify that the computation constant setting and the injectate volume are compatible. • To avoid repeating the injection procedure, correct the cardiac output (CO) value and the computation constant (CC) setting. To do so, use this formula: CO wrong × CC right ÷ CC wrong = CO right. Then reset the monitor for the next serial injection, using the correct computation constant.
	Catheter tip too far into pulmonary artery	• Check catheter placement by obtaining a pulmonary artery wedge pressure (PAWP) tracing. If the catheter is placed correctly, 1.25 to 1.5 cc of air will be necessary to obtain a PAWP tracing. • Reposition the catheter if necessary.
	Left to right ventricular septal defect	• Observe the PAWP tracing. A giant "V" wave indicates a ventricular septal defect and resultant incorrect cardiac output values. • Prepare to use another cardiac output monitoring method, such as the Fick method.
Cardiac output values deviating at least 10% from the mean (no pattern)	Arrhythmias, such as premature ventricular contractions and atrial fibrillation	• Observe the electrocardiogram monitor while monitoring cardiac output, and try to instill injectate during a period without arrhythmias. • Increase the number of serial injections to five or six, and average the values. • If the arrhythmias continue, notify the doctor.
	Catheter whip (turbulent, erratic waveform resulting from turbulence of blood circulating around intrusive catheter)	• Observe the waveforms, and reposition the catheter if necessary. • If catheter whip doesn't decrease spontaneously after the catheter is inserted or repositioned, increase the number of serial cardiac output determinations.
	Varying pulmonary artery baseline temperature (which causes drift during respiration)	• Obtain cardiac output values when respirations are steadier and less labored. • Minimize temperature variations by administering injectate during the same phase of the respiratory cycle each time you measure cardiac output. • Increase the number of serial injections.
	Variations in venous return (for example, from rapid bolus administration of drugs or fluids or from the patient's shivering, coughing, or restlessness)	• Avoid giving bolus injections of drugs or fluids just before measuring cardiac output. • If shivering accompanies a fever, notify the doctor. • Avoid measuring cardiac output until coughing or restlessness subsides.
	Inadequate signal-to-noise ratio	• To strengthen the signal, increase the injectate volume or lower the injectate temperature (for example, by using iced injectate for patients with hypothermia).
	Poor injection technique	• Observe the upstroke on the thermodilution curve to detect an error in injection technique. • Use two hands to deliver a bolus injection quickly and evenly.

MONITORING LEFT ATRIAL PRESSURE

Left atrial pressure (LAP) monitoring provides information about left ventricular function after open-heart surgery. A catheter inserted in the left atrium allows direct measurement of LAP. After being sutured to the pericardium, the catheter is drawn through a mediastinal incision on the chest wall and sutured to the skin.

LAP is created by blood volume in the left side of the heart and reflects the filling pressures in the left ventricle when the mitral valve is open. Unless the patient has mitral valve disease, LAP and the waveform produced during monitoring are reliable indicators of left ventricular end-diastolic pressure and, therefore, left ventricular function. Normal LAP ranges from 4 to 12 mm Hg. The LAP waveform resembles the pulmonary artery wedge pressure (PAWP) waveform.

LAP monitoring isn't performed routinely because pulmonary artery pressure (PAP) monitoring provides essential hemodynamic data with fewer risks. By monitoring PAP, you can approximate the LAP from the PAWP value. If the patient has a pulmonary artery catheter with a cardiac output port, you can measure cardiac output as well.

INDICATIONS

LAP monitoring is used primarily in heart transplant patients and in patients with left ventricular dysfunction who are undergoing cardiac surgery. It may also be used to evaluate treatment in patients with pulmonary hypertension, tricuspid or pulmonic valve disease, or abnormal cardiac anatomy. (In these patients, PAWP values may be unreliable indicators of left ventricular pressure.) Additionally, LAP monitoring may be initiated for patients with severe right ventricular failure who require infusion of prostaglandins and vasoconstrictors.

COMPLICATIONS

A major complication of LAP monitoring is systemic, cerebral, or coronary embolism, which may result from the introduction of air into the heart. (Using an air filter connected to a pressure transducer system can reduce the risk of this complication.) Another potential complication, bleeding at the insertion site may follow removal of the left atrial catheter and lead to life-threatening cardiac tamponade.

Setting up the system

Before the patient returns from the operating room, prepare a pressure transducer system with a fast flush device. You'll use heparin flush solution in the flush line. (To decrease the chance of flushing drugs and the risk of infection, this I.V. line should flow only to the left atrial catheter.)

Besides an I.V. pole, you'll need clean gloves, a gown, a face shield, an air filter, a 10-ml syringe, a monitor pressure cable, hypoallergenic tape, povidone-iodine ointment, sterile 4" × 4" gauze pads, a linen saver pad, a marking pen, and a carpenter's level or a ruler. You'll also need a monitor with LAP monitoring capabilities.

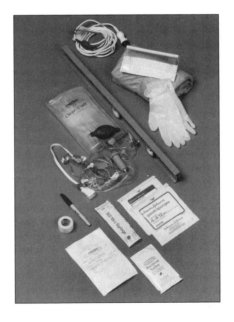
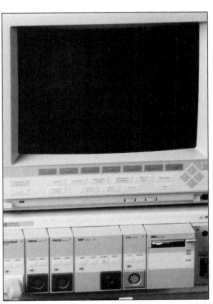

Cindy Tryniszewski, RN, MSN, Susan Galea, RN, MSN, CCRN, and *Cynthia Possanza, RN, MSN, CCRN,* contributed to this section. Ms. Tryniszewski is a clinical manager with Springhouse Corporation. Ms. Galea and Ms. Possanza are independent nurse consultants for Springhouse Corporation. The publisher thanks the following organizations for their help: *Medtronic, Inc.,* Minneapolis; *Medex, Inc.,* Hillard, Ohio; and *Hewlett-Packard Co.,* Andover, Mass.

After you assemble the equipment, unwrap the air filter. Then put on gloves and attach the air filter to the pressure transducer line at the end of the pressure transducer tubing. Secure all connections.

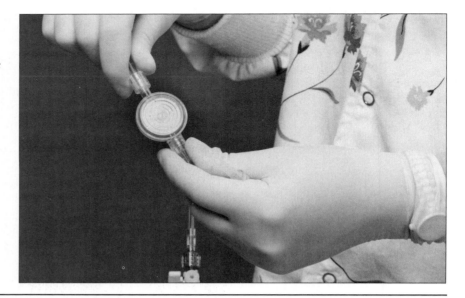

To expel air from the filter, remove the end cap on the filter, and squeeze the fast flush device (as shown). Let the filter fill completely with the heparin flush solution while you hold the filter upright to expel the air.

▶ *Clinical tip:* Completely saturate the filter with the flush solution by letting it rest for several minutes and then flushing it again.

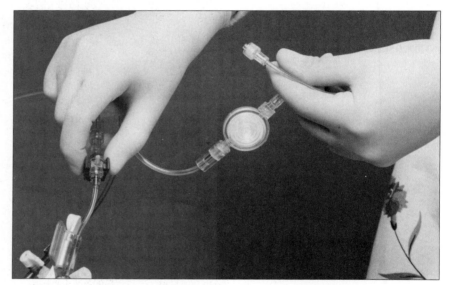

Now rotate the filter from front to back and check for air bubbles. If you see any, gently tap the filter and continue flushing.

▶ *Clinical tip:* Be sure to expel air from every part of the line. Otherwise, an air bubble may be forced into the patient's left atrium, causing an embolism.

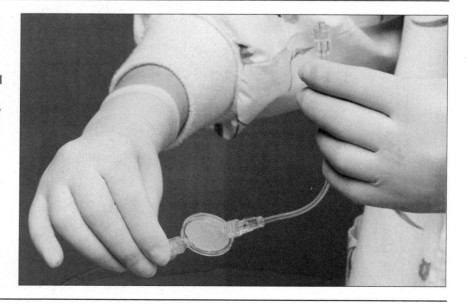

Take the prepared pressure transducer system and air filter to the patient's room and hang them on an I.V. pole. Insert the LAP module into the monitor if it's not already in place, and connect the monitor pressure cable to the LAP module. Then connect the transducer cable to the monitor pressure cable (as shown).

If you're using a manifold mount and it's not already in place, attach the mount to the I.V. pole and put the transducer into the mount.

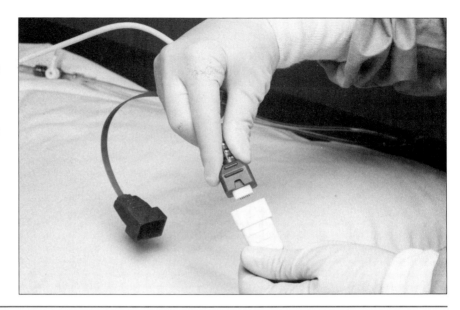

To ensure accurate pressure readings, position the transducer at the phlebostatic axis—the fourth intercostal space midway between the anterior and posterior chest wall. Position the transducer's air-fluid interface (located at the vent, or zero, port of the transducer's stopcock) level with this point (as shown).

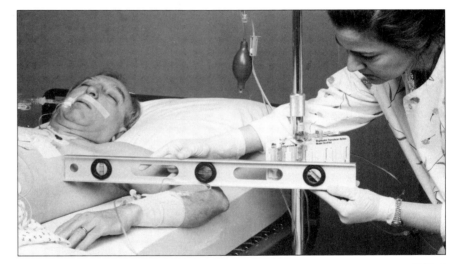

Use a marking pen to pinpoint the phlebostatic axis on the patient's chest or on a piece of tape applied to the patient's chest. This mark allows every nurse to use the same reference point when measuring LAP.

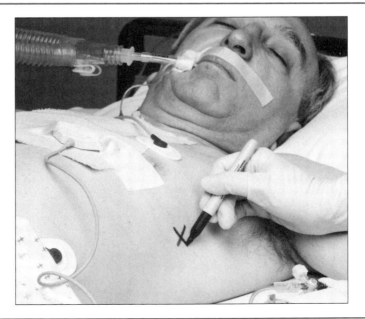

Turn the stopcock off to the patient, thereby opening the transducer to air. Then remove the cap from the vent port of the transducer (as shown).

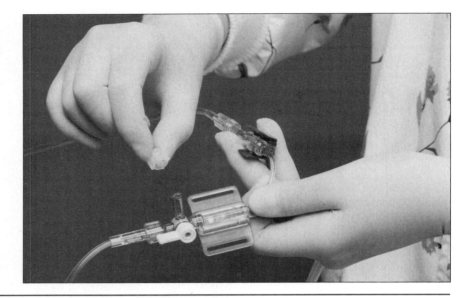

Following the manufacturer's manual, press the ZERO key on the monitor. Then press the CALIBRATE key. Keep in mind that some monitors require manipulation of a calibration key or knob, whereas others calibrate automatically. When you've finished zeroing, turn the stopcock on the transducer so that it's closed to air and open to the patient.

Continuing to follow the manufacturer's directions, select the appropriate mode and scale.

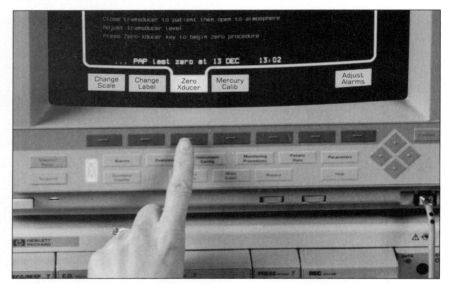

Before attaching the pressure transducer tubing to the left atrial catheter, put on clean gloves, a gown, and a face shield. Then remove the protective cap from the air filter at the end of the pressure transducer tubing. Be sure to turn the stopcock off to the patient before removing the cap from the left atrial catheter (as shown).

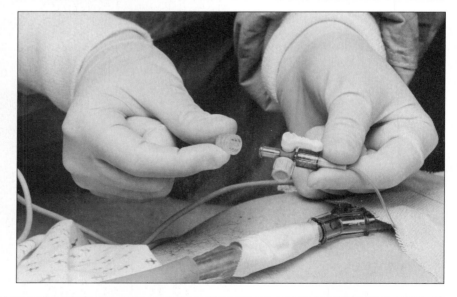

Place a linen-saver pad on the patient's chest. Then attach a 10-ml syringe to the open port of the stopcock. Pull back on the syringe to flush the stopcock and expel any air within the pressure tubing and stopcock.

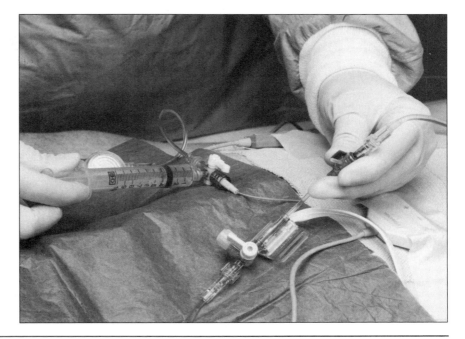

After you connect the tubing to the catheter, turn the stopcock to open the transducer to the patient. The patient's left atrial waveform should appear on the monitor.

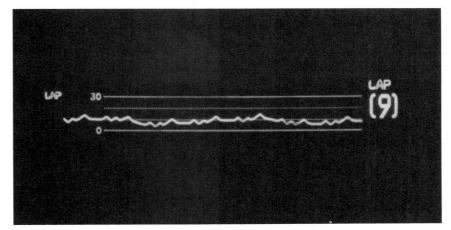

Review the alarm limits. If they need adjustment, set the high and low monitor alarms for the LAP limits determined by the doctor. Usually, you'll set the high alarm at 2 mm Hg above the baseline reading and the low alarm at 2 mm Hg below the baseline.

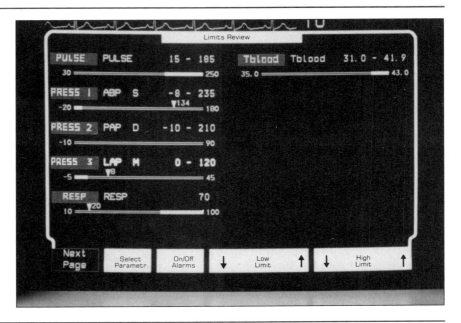

Alternatively, if the pressure transducer system and air filter were connected to the left atrial catheter in the operating room, connect the monitoring cable to the transducer (as shown). And turn the stopcock so that it's open to the patient.

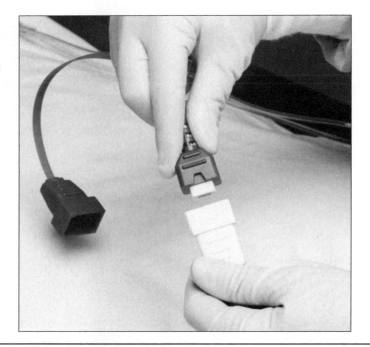

Once you've connected the patient to the pressure transducer system and the monitor, assess and care for the catheter site. Although the surgeon sutured the catheter to the skin, you can reinforce security by taping the catheter (as shown).

▶ *Clinical tip:* Alternatively, tape the air filter to a tongue blade and then to the patient's chest.

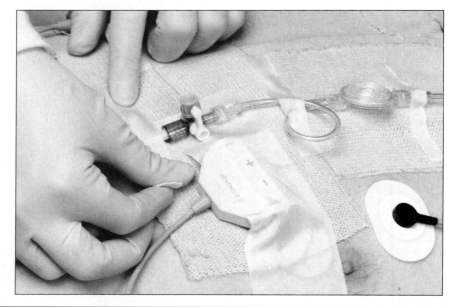

Taking the reading

Rezero the pressure transducer as described previously. Obtain the mean LAP measurement from the digital readout on the monitor screen (as shown). Note the LAP value at the end-expiration stage of respiration.

Then document the procedure and the first reading, noting the concentration of the heparin flush solution.

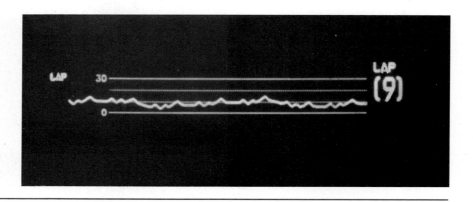

Continuously monitor the LAP waveform and pressure readings and compare them to other hemodynamic indices, such as cardiac output. Notify the doctor of any abnormal waveforms, including those revealing the catheter's migration to the left ventricle (as shown), damping, or a rise or fall of 2 mm Hg or more in the height of the A and V waves.

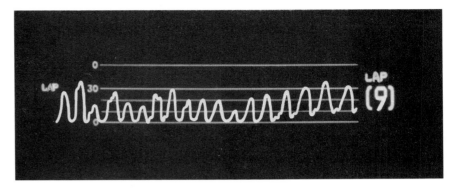

Document each reading as ordered or according to hospital protocol—usually hourly.

▶ ***Clinical tip:*** Remember that evaluating trends and changes in trends provides a more accurate picture of your patient's hemodynamic status and response to therapy than measuring isolated values alone.

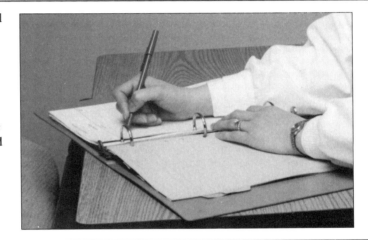

Discontinuing LAP monitoring

To assist with catheter removal, assemble the following equipment: sterile gloves, clean gloves, hypoallergenic tape, povidone-iodine ointment, a suture removal set, and sterile 4″ × 4″ gauze pads.

You'll also need equipment for observing universal precautions, including a face shield (or goggles and a mask), a gown, and gloves.

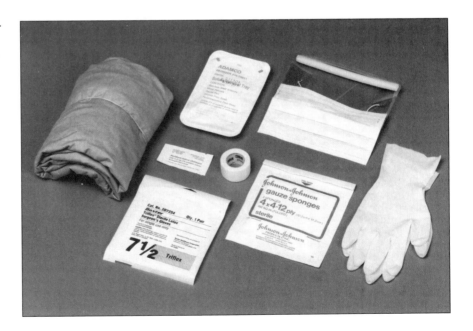

Explain the procedure to the patient. Then place him comfortably in the supine position with the head of the bed elevated 30 to 45 degrees. This decreases the risk of air embolism formation.

Turn off the monitor's LAP alarm while taking care not to turn off other alarms. Then put on the clean gloves, gown, and face shield.

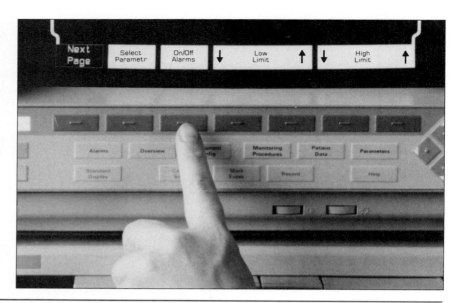

Close the flow clamp on the tubing of the pressurized heparin flush solution.

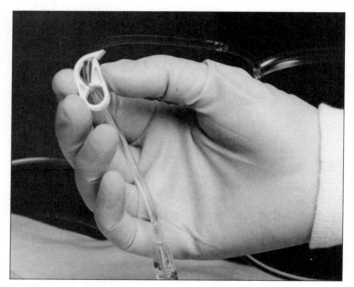

Turn the stopcock closest to the patient off to the patient.

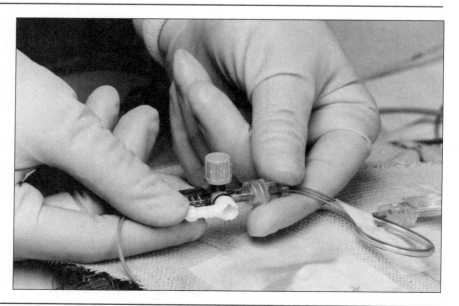

Remove the dressing. Then remove and discard your gloves and put on a pair of sterile gloves.

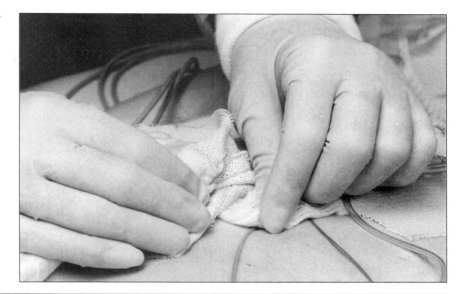

Immediately after the doctor cuts the sutures that hold the catheter to the patient's skin and removes the catheter, apply direct pressure to the exit site with sterile 4″ × 4″ gauze pads. Continue applying manual pressure for 10 minutes to prevent hemorrhage.

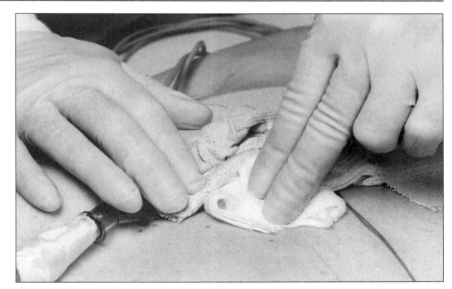

Once you're sure that the bleeding has stopped, apply povidone-iodine ointment to the site and cover it with dry, sterile 4″ × 4″ gauze pads. Tape the dressing in place.

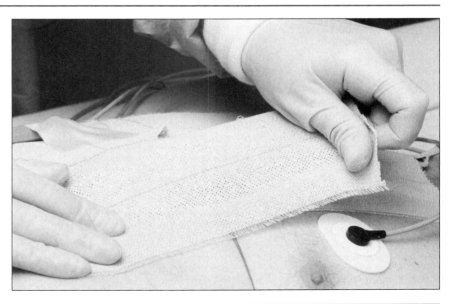

Check the catheter to make sure that it's intact. If you see evidence of breakage or other damage, notify the doctor immediately and save the catheter for the doctor to examine. Otherwise, dispose of the equipment according to hospital policy.

Auscultate the patient's breath and heart sounds and check vital signs and chest tube drainage every 15 minutes for the first hour, every 30 minutes for the next hour, and every hour thereafter or according to hospital protocol. Notify the doctor if you detect a significant increase or decrease in chest tube drainage or abnormal vital signs.

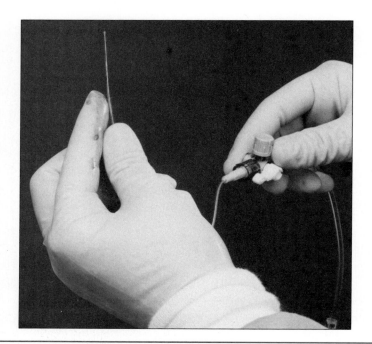

About 1 hour after catheter removal, check the dressing for signs of bleeding and the exit site for signs of a hematoma. If you observe such signs, apply pressure to the site and notify the doctor. If you don't observe any bleeding or a hematoma, redress the site as you dressed it initially.

As ordered, arrange for a chest X-ray about 1 hour after catheter removal to assess for cardiac tamponade. Then document the procedure.

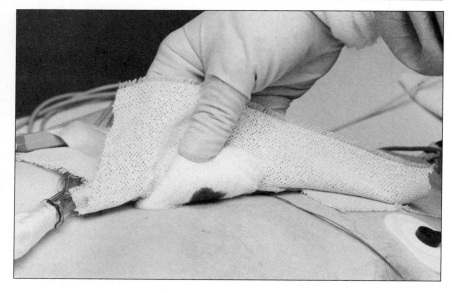

INSIGHTS AND INTERPRETATIONS

Understanding LAP waveforms

The normal left atrial pressure (LAP) waveform reflects low pressure. Similar to the pulmonary artery wedge pressure waveform, it has two positive deflections and consists of four distinct components: the A wave, the X descent, the V wave, and the Y descent.

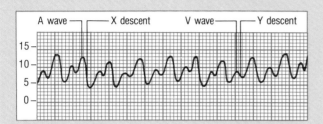

The first positive deflection, the *A wave,* represents left atrial contraction (also referred to as left atrial kick), which forces blood from the left atrium through the mitral valve and into the left ventricle.

After the left atrium contracts and before the mitral valve closes, the pressure in the left atrium falls and the waveform begins a downward slope, identified as the *X descent.*

During ventricular systole, the left atrium fills with blood and the mitral valve closes. At this point, the second positive deflection—the *V wave*—appears as the closed mitral valve bulges into the left atrium.

At the end of ventricular systole, the pressure in the left atrium decreases. This is represented as a downward slope of the V wave called the *Y descent.*

Abnormal LAP waveforms

Various conditions can produce abnormal LAP waveforms with the following features:

• *Absent A wave.* In atrial fibrillation, no A wave will appear in the LAP waveform because the atria only quiver and the left atrium doesn't contract. The mean LAP will increase in atrial fibrillation.

• *Prominent A wave.* Any condition that increases pressure or volume in the left atrium during atrial contraction will produce a prominent A wave. In patients with complete heart block or atrioventricular dissociation, the left atrium may contract against a closed mitral valve at times. The result: increasing LAP, which causes a prominent A wave.

In patients with mitral stenosis, the narrowing of the mitral valve obstructs blood flow from the left atrium to the left ventricle. To pump blood effectively to the left ventricle, the LAP must be high enough to force the blood through the stenotic valve. If the patient is in normal sinus rhythm, the LAP waveform will reveal a prominent A wave.

• *Prominent V wave.* This waveform abnormality may result from any condition that causes an increase in left atrial volume or pressure during left ventricular systole. In mitral insufficiency, for example, the incompetent mitral valve allows blood from the left ventricle to flow back into the left atrium during systole. This results in a prominent V wave unless the left atrium has enlarged enough to accommodate the regurgitated volume.

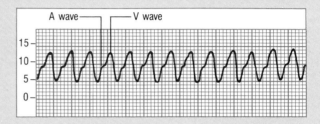

Evaluating the data

Before interpreting the data from the LAP waveforms, always remember to take pressure readings on the monitor's mean mode. Also, be sure to take readings at the end-expiration stage of respiration. Normally, a patient's LAP will fall during inspiration because of the drop in intrathoracic pressure and will rise to baseline during expiration.

Mean LAP ranges between 4 and 12 mm Hg. If your monitoring system doesn't automatically display the mean LAP value, use this equation:

$$\text{Mean LAP} = \frac{(\text{LAP diastolic} \times 2) + (\text{LAP systolic})}{3}$$

Decreased LAP

Expect LAP to decline as a result of hypovolemia from reduced fluid intake, postoperative hemorrhage, and postoperative rewarming that causes vasodilation.

Increased LAP

Expect LAP to rise from such conditions as mitral stenosis, tachyarrhythmias, a noncompliant left ventricle, and hypervolemia. In *mitral stenosis,* obstructed blood flow from the left atrium to the left ventricle increases left atrial volume and pressure. In *tachyarrhythmias,* the left ventricle's inability to eject a normal volume of blood raises LAP. In a *noncompliant left ventricle,* decreased myocardial contractility reduces blood ejection from the left ventricle, resulting in increased left ventricular pressure and LAP. In *hypervolemia,* increased fluid volume returning to the heart augments pressure within the heart.

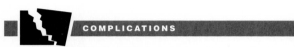

COMPLICATIONS

Managing hazards of LAP monitoring

PROBLEM AND SIGNS	POSSIBLE CAUSES	NURSING INTERVENTIONS
Clotted catheter tip • Damped or straight waveform on the monitor	• Localized coagulation • Blood clot or air bubble • Sluggish flush solution flow • Insufficient heparin in flush solution	• Notify the doctor. He may attempt to aspirate the clot to prevent its release into the general circulation. Once he removes the clot, he may flush the catheter; if the clot resists removal, he'll usually remove the catheter.
Blood loss • Bloody dressing • Blood flowing from disconnected line	• Disconnected line • Dislodged catheter	• If the line disconnects, turn the stopcock closest to the patient off to the patient, and replace the equipment. • If the catheter pulls out, apply direct pressure to the site and notify the doctor. Also notify him if blood loss is great and vital signs change.
Hemorrhage • Increased sanguineous drainage from mediastinal chest tubes • Any or all of the following: hypotension, tachycardia, irritability, oliguria, pallor, and cool, clammy skin • Decreased pulmonary artery wedge pressure, decreased left atrial pressure (LAP)	• Bleeding from insertion site into mediastinum	• Notify the doctor immediately. • Check the patient's vital signs. • Administer fluids, blood products, and oxygen as prescribed. • In cases of inadequate gas exchange, prepare the patient for intubation. • If bleeding continues, prepare the patient for surgical intervention.
Embolism (air embolism or cerebral, coronary, or systemic thromboembolism) • Fall in blood pressure • Rise in central venous pressure (CVP) • Weak, rapid pulse • Cyanosis • Loss of consciousness or change in level of consciousness	• Air in tubing • Loose connections	• Notify the doctor and monitor vital signs. • Place the patient in Trendelenburg's position on his left side. If air has entered the heart chambers, this position may keep the air in the heart and out of circulation. • Check the line for a leak or a disconnection. • If the line disconnects, don't rejoin it. Replace the part with sterile equipment. Meanwhile, turn the stopcock off to the patient or clamp the line with a rubber-shod hemostat. • Administer oxygen if ordered. • Alert the doctor if you detect any systemic abnormalities.
Systemic infection • Sudden rise in patient's body temperature and pulse rate • Chills and shaking • Blood pressure changes	• Poor aseptic technique or contamination of equipment during manufacture, storage, or use	• Look for other sources of infection first. Obtain specimens of urine, sputum, and blood for culture as ordered. • Notify the doctor, who will probably discontinue the line and send the catheter tip for culture and sensitivity tests. • Administer antibiotics as prescribed.
Endocarditis • Intermittent fever, night sweats • Loud, regurgitant heart murmur • Weakness, fatigue • Weight loss, anorexia • Arthralgia	• Poor aseptic technique or contamination of equipment during manufacture, storage, or use	• Notify the doctor, who may discontinue the line. • Administer antibiotics as prescribed.
Catheter displacement • Ventricular arrhythmias • Heightened V waves • Absent valve click in a patient with a prosthetic mitral valve	• Catheter improperly sutured or taped to skin	• Notify the doctor if you think that the catheter moved; prepare to assist with catheter repositioning or removal. • Administer antiarrhythmic agents as prescribed.
Cardiac tamponade • Reduced cardiac output • Muffled heart sounds • Pulsus paradoxus • Neck vein distention • Reduced arterial blood pressure • Markedly elevated CVP or an equalization of CVP and pulmonary artery pressure • Decreased voltage reflected in the QRS complex • Sudden increase or decrease in chest tube drainage	• An accumulation of blood or fluid in pericardial sac	• Notify the doctor, who may order surgery. • Assess and document electrocardiogram rhythm patterns, vital signs, mental status, heart and breath sounds, and urine output. • Initiate I.V. volume therapy, as prescribed, with fluids and volume expanders. • Administer oxygen if ordered. • Administer inotropic agents as prescribed. • Begin resuscitative measures if necessary.

Caring for the patient with a left atrial catheter

During the insertion of a left atrial catheter and during the critical postoperative period after its insertion, you'll need to monitor your patient's hemodynamic status, ensure that the monitoring equipment is working effectively and safely, and prevent complications. Here are some guidelines.

Monitor hemodynamic status
• Measure and record left atrial pressure (LAP) at least hourly. Obtain the mean LAP at end expiration.
• Take your patient's vital signs at least hourly. To ensure accurate interpretation of values, take LAP readings at the same time that you measure the patient's blood pressure, heart rate, central venous pressure, pulmonary artery pressure, and urine output.
• Monitor the patient's LAP waveform. Watch for any increase in the height of the baseline V waves and a rise of 2 mm Hg or more in pressure. If you detect such an increase, notify the doctor.

Ensure effective operation
• To keep the left atrial catheter line and connecting tubing patent, make sure that a pressurized heparin flush solution continuously flows through the line. Check the flow rate hourly and maintain it at 3 to 4 ml/hour. Add more heparin to the solution if ordered.
• Balance and calibrate the pressure transducer at least once every 8 hours.
• Continuously monitor the LAP waveform, the electrocardiogram, and other pressure tracings. If you notice waveform damping, notify the doctor. Consult the manufacturer's manual as needed.
• If the patient has a prosthetic mitral valve, auscultate for the valve click sound. Notify the doctor immediately if you don't hear this sound; it may indicate that the left atrial catheter has slipped through the prosthetic valve.

Prevent complications
• Review and maintain sterile technique.
• Change the dressing at the insertion site every 24 hours or as recommended by hospital protocol. Check for redness, drainage, or broken sutures. If you detect any of these problems, notify the doctor immediately.
• Watch for bleeding from the insertion site (and, possibly, hemorrhage or cardiac tamponade if bleed-

ing affects the pericardial sac). This may occur if the catheter's size and position were inappropriate for the patient. To minimize complications that may accompany bleeding, check the patient's prothrombin and partial thromboplastin times. Also check the platelet count, which should be higher than 60,000/mm^3. If any results are abnormal, notify the doctor.
• Avoid contaminating the catheter site when bathing the patient.
• Don't rejoin any portion of a disconnected line. Instead, replace the portion with sterile equipment.
• Never infuse any I.V. fluids or medications other than the prescribed flush solution through the left atrial catheter line. If the catheter clogs, don't flush it or attempt to aspirate the occlusion. Notify the doctor immediately.
• Change the components of the system as recommended by hospital policy. For example, change a flush solution bag before it empties or every 24 hours. Change the pressure bag holding the flush solution at least once every 24 hours and the pressure tubing and the filter once every 48 hours.
• Frequently check the catheter connections and the insertion site. Check the taped connections for security, and make sure that the tape holding the catheter in place remains secure.
• Be alert for air bubbles in the system. If you detect any, attempt to expel the air. If you're unsuccessful, notify the doctor immediately. Always expel all air from the line before attaching it to the left atrial catheter.
• Measure and record chest tube drainage hourly. Notify the doctor of a significant increase or decrease in sanguineous drainage, which may indicate hemorrhage or developing cardiac tamponade.
• Monitor the patient and his waveform for signs of ventricular arrhythmias, and notify the doctor at once should any occur.
• Auscultate the patient's heart at least once every 4 hours or whenever you see a significant change in the LAP value or waveform. Notify the doctor of significant changes.
• Keep the patient on bed rest at all times.
• Be sure to arrange for a daily X-ray of the patient's chest to verify correct placement of the left atrial catheter.

Solving LAP monitoring problems

PROBLEM	POSSIBLE CAUSES	NURSING INTERVENTIONS
Damped waveform Interference with transmission of the physiologic signal to the transducer	• Air in the system	• Check the entire system for air, including the tubing and transducer diaphragm. If air is present, flush it from the system through a stopcock port. Do not flush fluid into the patient.
	• Loose connections • Occluded catheter tip	• Check and tighten all connections. • Notify the doctor, who may try to aspirate the occlusion. If successful, he'll flush the line to restore patency; if unsuccessful, he'll remove the line.
	• Catheter tip resting against the left atrium wall • Kinked tubing • Inadequately inflated pressure bag	• Reposition the patient. • Unkink the tubing. • Inflate the pressure bag to 300 mm Hg.
False-high pressure reading Values are higher than the patient's normal values with no significant change in baseline clinical findings. Before responding to the high reading, recheck the system for accuracy.	• Improper calibration • Transducer placed below the level of the phlebostatic axis • Kinked catheter • Occluded catheter tip	• Recalibrate the system. • Reposition the transducer so that it's level with the phlebostatic axis. • Unkink the catheter. • Notify the doctor, who may try to aspirate the occlusion. If he's successful, he'll flush the line to restore patency; if he's unsuccessful, he'll remove the catheter.
	• Catheter tip resting against the left atrium wall • Small air bubbles in the tubing closest to the patient	• Reposition the patient. • Flush air bubbles from the system through a stopcock port. Do not flush fluid into the patient.
False-low pressure reading Values are lower than the patient's normal values with no significant changes in baseline clinical findings. Before responding to the low reading, recheck the system for accuracy.	• Improper calibration • Transducer placed above the level of the phlebostatic axis • Loose connections • Kinked catheter • Catheter tip resting against the left atrium wall • Large air bubble close to the transducer	• Recalibrate the system. • Reposition the transducer so that it's level with the phlebostatic axis. • Check and tighten all connections. • Unkink the catheter. • Reposition the patient. • Reprime the transducer.
Artifact Waveforms are erratic or form unrecognizable patterns.	• Electrical interference • Patient movement	• Check electrical equipment in the area. • Instruct the patient to lie quietly while you read the monitor.
Drifting waveform Waveform floats above and below the baseline.	• Temperature change in the flush solution • Kinked or compressed monitor cable	• Allow temperature of the flush solution to stabilize. • Check the cable and fix the kink or compression.
Absent waveform	• No power supply • Loose connections • Stopcock turned off to the patient	• Turn on the power. • Check and tighten all connections. • Properly position the stopcock. Be sure that the pressure transducer line is open to the catheter.
	• Transducer disconnected from the monitor module • Occluded catheter tip	• Reconnect the transducer to the monitor module. • Notify the doctor, who may try to aspirate the occlusion. If he's successful, he'll flush the line to restore patency; if he's unsuccessful, he'll remove the line.
	• Catheter tip resting against the left atrium wall	• Reposition the patient.

INDEX